G000277391

STRESS RELIEF FOR WOMEN

JANET WRIGHT

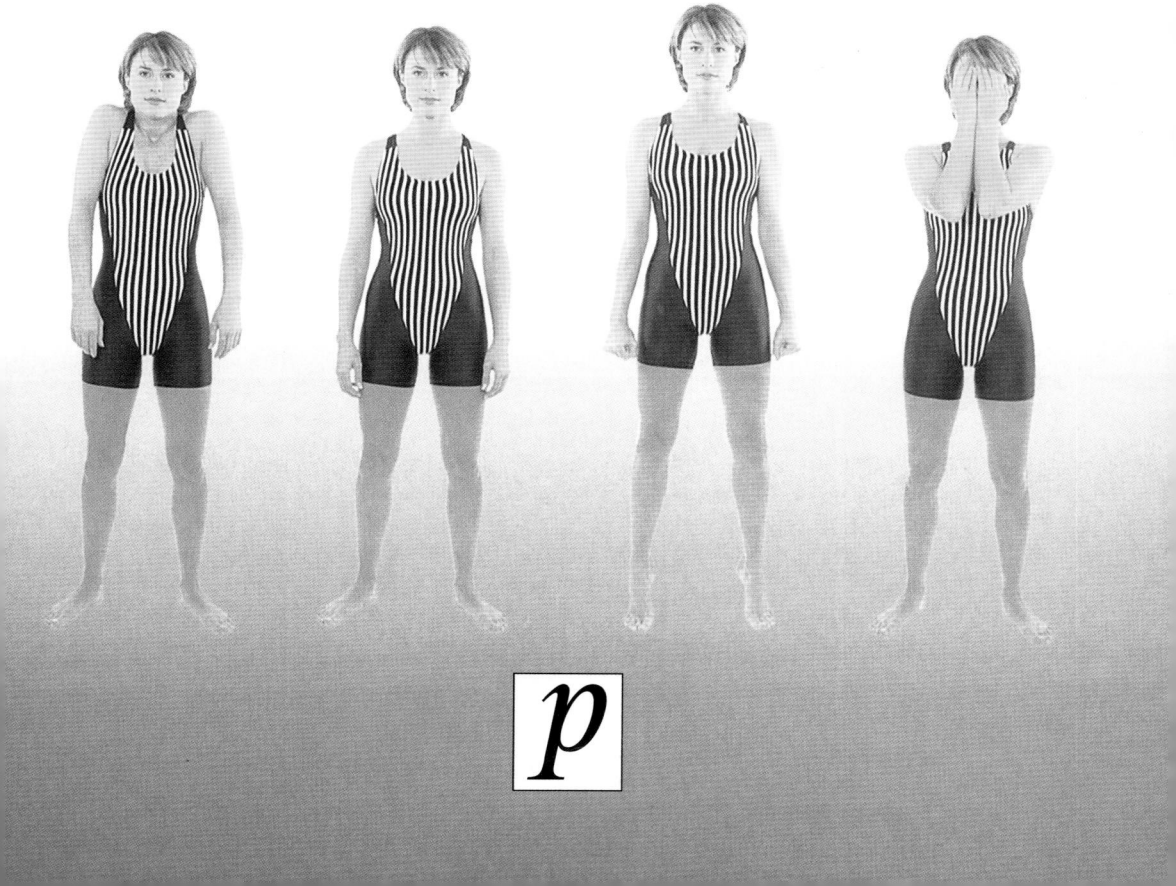

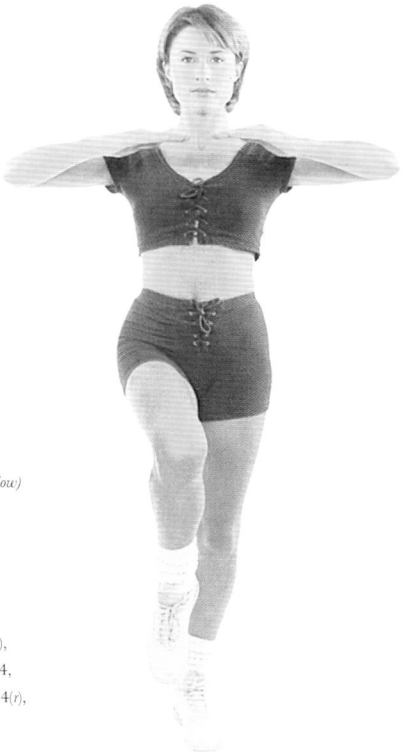

This is a Parragon Book
This edition published in 2002

Parragon
Queen Street House
4 Queen Street
Bath BA1 1HE, UK

Copyright © Parragon 1997

Designed, produced and packaged by
Touchstone
Old Chapel Studio, Plain Road, Marden,
Tonbridge, Kent TN12 9LS, United Kingdom

All rights reserved. No part of this publication may be reproduced, stored in a retrieval system, or transmitted in any way or by any means, electronic, mechanical, photocopying, recording or otherwise, without the prior permission of the copyright holder.

ISBN 0-75257-754-9

Printed in Spain

Photographic credits:
(Abbreviations: r = right, l = left, t = top, b = below)

The publishers would like to thank the following for permission to reproduce their photographs:

Telegraph Colour Library: Pages 7, 8(*b*), 11(*tl*), 12, 13, 14, 15(*t, r*), 16, 17, 18, 22(*l*), 24, 25(*bl, br*), 36, 45, 56, 64(*b*), 72, 82(*r*), 83(*r*), 84(*r*), 85, 86(*l*), 90, 91(*t*).

The Image Bank: Pages 84(*l*), 91(*b*).

Touchstone: Pages 11(*br*), 15(*l, br*), 22(*t, br*), 23(*tl, tr*), 26(*b*), 69(*t*), 71(*tl*), 73(*t*), 76(*r*), 77, 79, 80(*br*), 81(*r*).

All other pictures © Parragon Publishing

With thanks to Pinpoint Photography and Peter Pugh-Cook for all commissioned photographs.

Disclaimer
The exercises, and therapies detailed in this book are suitable for normally healthy adults. the author, publisher, their servants or agents cannot accept responsibility for loss or damage suffered by individuals as a result of following any advise in this book. It is strongly recommended that individuals suffering from, or with a history of, high blood pressure, heart disease or any other medical condition, undertake demanding physical exertion only after seeking professional advice from their doctor.

STRESS RELIEF
FOR WOMEN

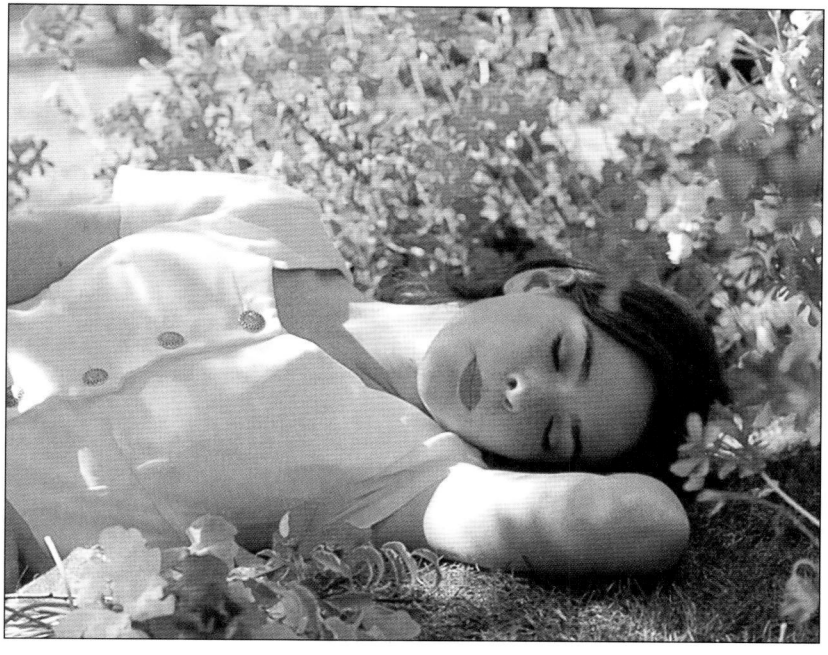

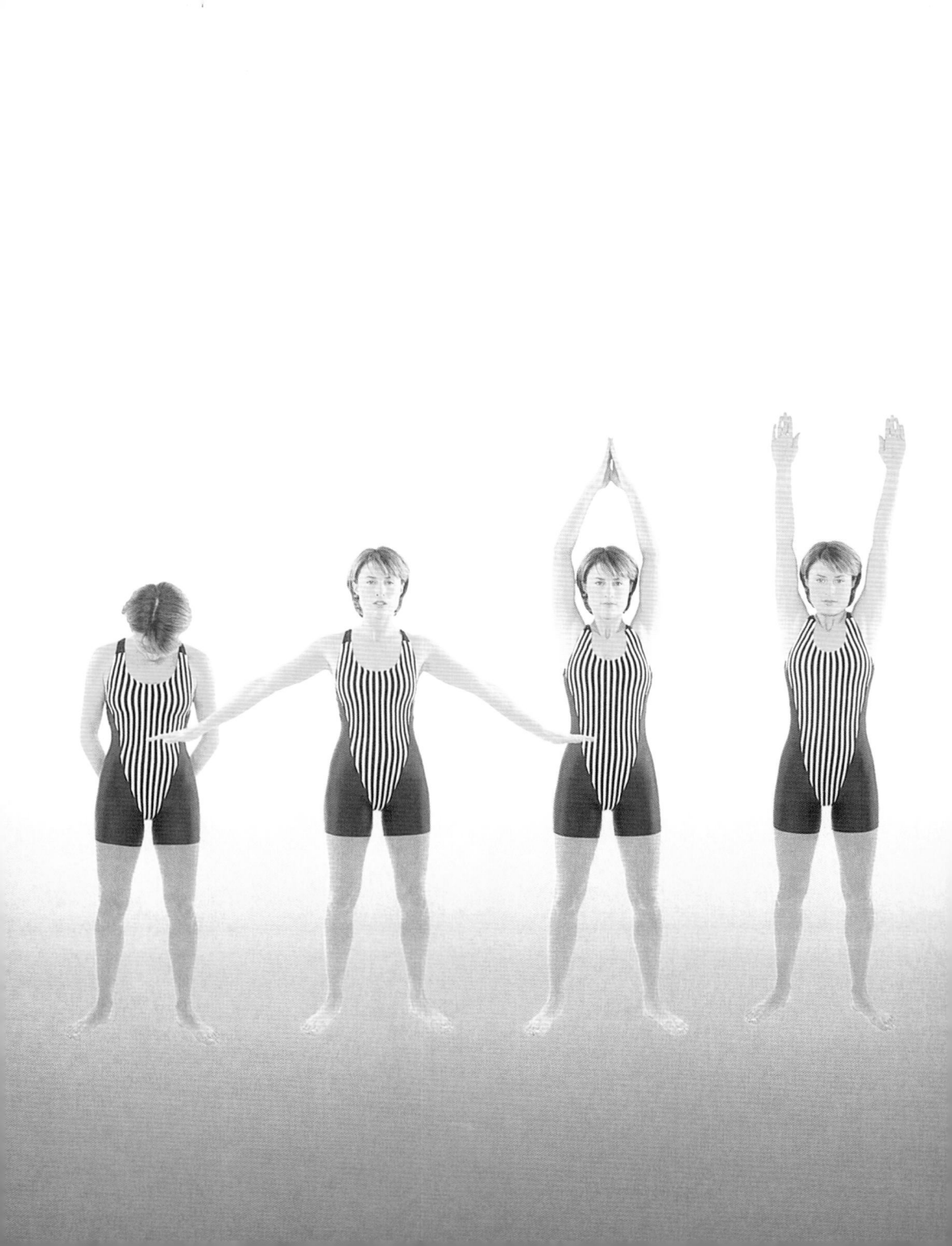

Contents

What Causes Stress? 6
The Unrelaxers 8
Hormonal Upheaval 10
Peaceful Pregnancy 12
Relax? With Kids Like Mine? 14
Moving With The Change 16
Coping With Pain 18
Stress Relief First Aid 20
Eat to Stay on Top 22
Organize to Avoid Stress 24
A Safe Place to Relax 26
Breathe Your Troubles Away 28
Taking It From The Top 30
Foot-To-Head Relaxation 32
Make Your Own Relaxation Tape 34
Massage – The Healing Touch 36
Massage Yourself 38
Shiatsu – Pressing a Point 40
Aromatherapy – Healing Scents 42
Reflexology – Body and Sole 44
The Alexander Technique 46
Yoga – Your Flexible Friend 48
T'ai Chi – Chinese Serenity 50
Exercise – Dump Your Stress 52
Stretch – Relax Like a Cat 54
Walk Away From Your Troubles 56
Belly Dance – Eastern Promise 58
Autogenic Training 60
Meditation 62
Mindfulness 64
Moving Meditation 66
Hypnosis – Reach Your Inner Self 68
Self-Hypnosis 70
Colour Therapy 72
Voice & Music Therapy 74
Herbalism – Power of Plants 76
Homeopathy – Like Cures Like 78
Flower Remedies 80
Spas & Beauty Therapy 82
Bath Delights 84
Planning a Relaxation Day 86
On The Day 88
The Most Important Thing 90
Shopping to Relax 92
More Information 94
Index 96

What Causes Stress?

The modern Western way of life could have been designed to cause early heart attacks. But not many of us have the chance to go and live on a tropical island – and we'd probably miss a lot if we did. The more practical answer is to make the most of living here and cut down on the stress.

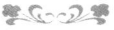

Feeling stressed doesn't mean you're neurotic. It's a perfectly natural response to events that threaten our safety. At the first sign of danger, our whole metabolism switches onto a war footing. We stop digesting food or making internal repairs. Our bodies are flooded with adrenaline and other emergency hormones to rush oxygen around the body and release quick-energy fuel into the bloodstream. For a few minutes we're the strongest and fastest we can possibly be – just long enough to spear that wolf or run away from that landslide.

Mmm, that's the trouble. The stress response was designed for a time when danger was deadly but brief. It's just as good today, for the record-breaking leap to stop a toddler pulling a hot saucepan down on her head, but more often that heart-thudding rush happens when we're stuck in a traffic jam or faced with a bill we can't pay. Unused, the stress hormones linger in our bodies, wreaking havoc on our health.

These days we tend to have long-term problems. We want some control over our lives, but things are changing all around us and sometimes we're swept along with the tide. Jobs are insecure, marriage is no longer a life-long commitment, our food and environment are increasingly polluted, we work longer hours than ever before, it's hard to make ends meet and the world seems full of dangers to our children. Relationships and family problems add to the list of worries. We feel responsible for everyone's well-being but powerless to make everything all right, every time. A recipe for stress.

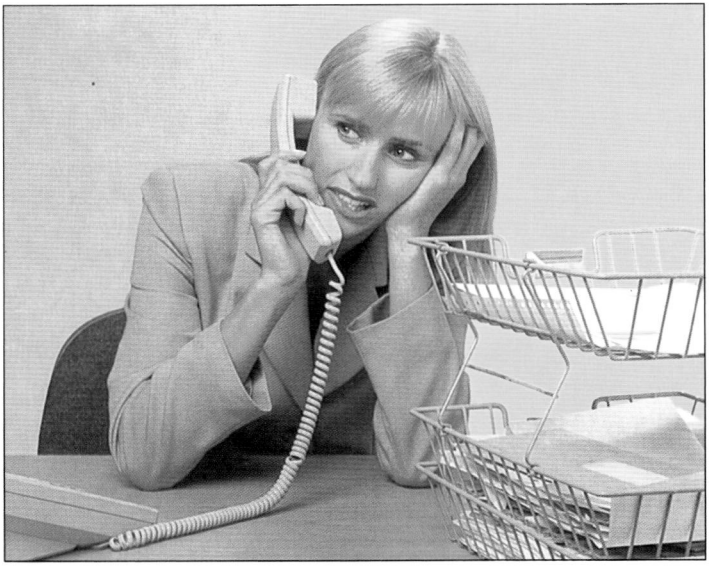

Learning To Relax

Do we really need to learn how to relax? Look at a cat asleep by the fire – no one taught it how to flop into instant sleep or wake up with a long and sensuous stretch, ready for anything. But when did you last feel so relaxed? The trouble is, human beings have a far more complicated life than cats.

Somewhere between inventing the wheel and weaving the Internet we've forgotten most of what cats know about staying healthy. Babies still know – but as we go out into the speedy, competitive adult world, it all slips away. Until we start feeling exhausted, troubled by niggling pains or unaccountably near to tears, we don't even realize we've lost something we need.

◁ Working longer hours than ever before, we find ourselves under a great deal of stress.

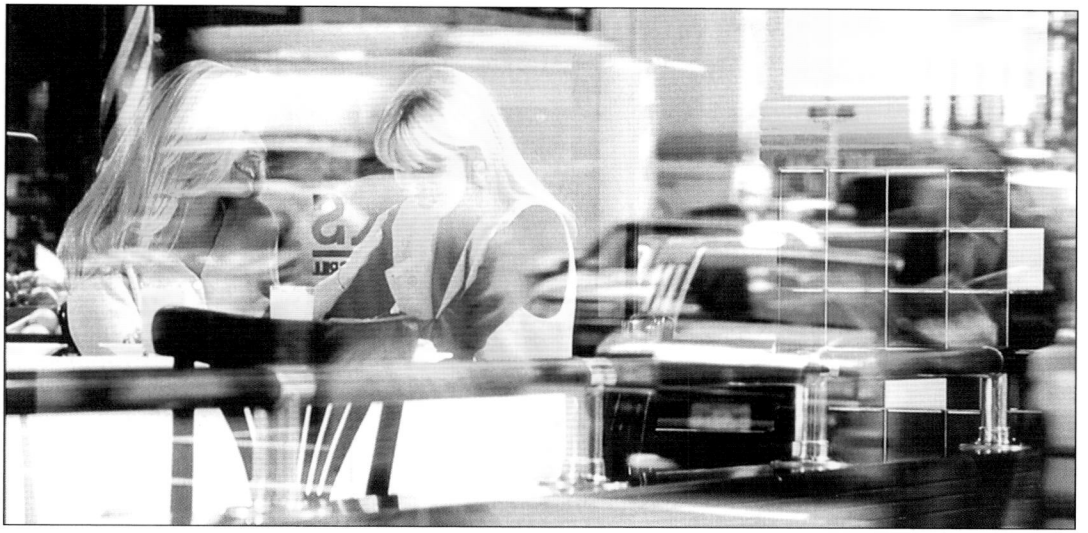

△ *Relaxation should not be yet another task to fit into an already crowded day.*

The techniques in this book are just as good for either sex. But women often tend to have more responsibilities and less time or money to spend on their own needs. Though most of us now do a paid job as well as running a home, the figures show we still do almost all the housework and childcare. An ever-increasing number are doing the whole lot by themselves. Women are brought up to care about everyone else and, when time's at a premium, looking after themselves is the easiest task to drop.

So some of the tips in this book are 10-second lifesavers – for moments of crisis or when you simply can't take the break you need.

Relaxation is a powerful medicine. It speeds recovery from all kinds of illnesses and, better still, can help prevent them in the first place. It magics away the pain caused by muscles we didn't even realize were tensed up like fists. It relieves stress, with its many and varied physical manifestations from indigestion to heart disorders. It keeps us young, not only smoothing out the lines etched into our faces but giving us years more healthy, active life. It brings back the sort of energy we used to take for granted – how often have you watched children playing and thought 'Was I ever as lively as that?'. In short, it makes life a lot more enjoyable.

Most of us think we could relax perfectly well if we had more time. Yet when there is time, what do we do? Collapse in front of the television, even when there's nothing we want to watch, because we're too tired to do anything we'd enjoy more or there's no one to look after the children. Then, disturbed by the news and frazzled by canned laughter, we sleep badly and wake up more tired than ever.

A week on a health farm might do us all good. But that's not the only route to relaxation, by a long way. Take your pick from techniques that are sociable or solitary, a two-minute pick-me-up or a two-hour ritual, quick to learn or part of a long-term investment in your future, recommended by doctors or taught by spiritual leaders, invented for modern needs or as old as time. This book looks at dozens of options, especially ones that are cheap and simple. Relaxation isn't yet another task to fit into a crowded day. It's about finding ways you enjoy that work for you.

How to use this book

Almost all the techniques in this book can be tried at home, so it's full of easy exercises and do-it-yourself tips. Some of them will be all you need. Others, if you like them, you can go on to learn more fully in a class or buy a book on the subject.

Where no exercises are given, it's because the technique really needs to be taught personally by a trained expert. In the 'Where Do I Go From Here?' pages at the end there's a list of organizations and books for further information.

The Unrelaxers

We've all got favourite ways of relaxing, but some are more effective than others and some aren't really relaxing at all. Let's be honest – flopping in front of the television can be just the job after a day spent running after children and speeding round the shops. But edge-of-the-seat games shows and horror films can leave your heart pounding like a woodpecker. And if you've spent an equally tiring day sitting at a desk, more sitting is just what you don't need.

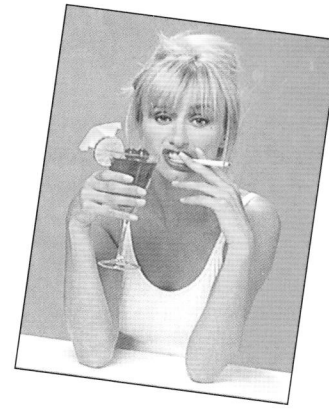

△ *Can we really relax with stimulants?*

For many women, a coffee or cigarette break is the only chance they get to stop working. But caffeine and nicotine are stimulants, not relaxers. The short break is actually to 'unrelax', to take chemicals on board that will help you stay alert a bit longer. They do just the same when you've finished work, though, and are trying to wind down. They are addictive, so having one is a relief because it stops the craving.

But while sitting down to a familiar ritual can be relaxing in itself, the caffeine and nicotine whizzing round your bloodstream keep everything hyped up. Even tea contains some caffeine. Herbal teas, or the beverages sold in health food shops, are a better bet for relaxing.

Alcohol is famous for helping people relax – often more than they intended to. But though it can ease stress, unknot tense muscles and bring on sleep, the benefits are only temporary – you'll breathe shallowly and wake up early. Beware, too, if you start finding you can't relax without it.

Not all drugs are equal, of course. A drink or a couple of coffees a day shouldn't do any harm unless you're pregnant or have been warned off by your doctor. Some researchers even recommend a glass of wine a day to keep the heart healthy. Tobacco, on the other hand, offers no benefits of any kind. It's harmful even in small amounts and – never mind dying young – causes more boring, painful, totally avoidable ill-health than anything else in the Western world. Relaxing with a cigarette is like trying to sleep on a bed of nails – it causes stressful reactions such as speeding up your heart, so the body can't relax deeply. It's expensive too, saving the

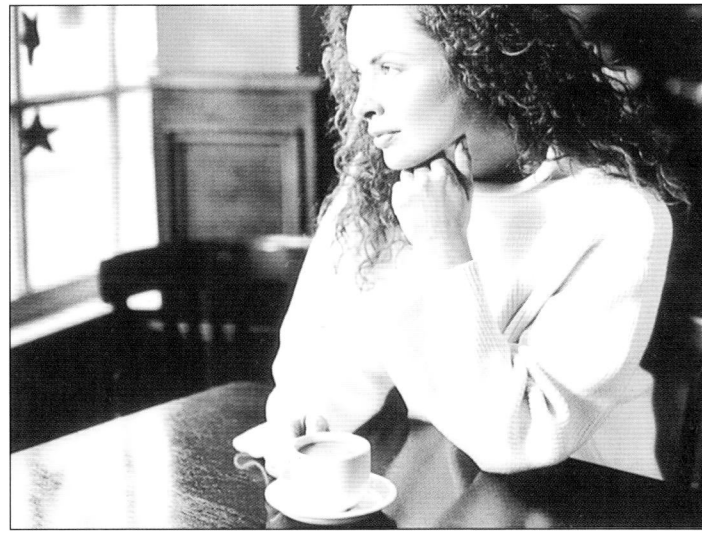

△ *The caffeine in coffee and tea may do more to wake you up than to help you relax.*

cost of a packet of cigarettes a day will pay for a genuinely relaxing weekly treat. If you're worried about putting on weight, healthy eating and exercise will keep it off.

Overeating is another false friend when you're under stress. Don't feel guilty, just find more helpful ways of being kind to yourself when you need it.

Tranquillizers may seem the only answer when you're desperate, but these addictive drugs only help for a short time, if at all. After that, they cause more damage than they could ever have cured. If you're at the end of your tether, ring the Samaritans – listed in your local phone book – or ask your doctor to refer you for counselling or to put you in touch with one of the self-help groups set up by fellow-sufferers for all kinds of problems. These can also give sympathetic, practical advice if you're already hooked and need help coming off.

Standing up to stress

When something makes you feel stressed, there are three ways of reacting:

1. Change things outside, by taking action to solve the problem.

2. Change things inside, by accepting what's happening and coming to terms with it.

3. Do neither, and worry helplessly.

Needless to say, the first course of action is best, whether it's joining an environmental action group or refusing to clean up after everyone. Some things can't be changed so, option 2, you simply have to live with them – any energy you put into resenting them is wasted. Often, though, you can compromise with a mixture of 1 and 2.

Take money, for example – that prime source of worry. You can try to earn more or spend less. Cut up credit cards and find new pleasures that don't cost anything, until the wheel of fortune turns back in your favour.

Contact anyone you owe money (especially if they own your home) and arrange to pay in manageable installments.

Take whatever steps you can to protect yourself and your family, stay out of any more debt, look after your health, learn new skills that could earn extra cash.

And then stop worrying. Hard to do, yes, but not impossible. Meditation and breathing techniques are a big help here, creating a feeling of peace and calmness. And like any exercise, they get easier the more you practice.

Worry is worse than useless – its paralysing effects stop people doing anything constructive. It stops you enjoying what you've got. And it can cause a host of problems of its own, such as phobias and panic attacks.

Learning to relax clears the mind and frees up energy, making it easier to find solutions. The only answer is:

- Relax.
- Think what to do.
- Do it.
- Get on with your life.

KEEP WORRIES IN THEIR PLACE

If you can't stop fretting over a problem:

- Make an appointment with it. Every afternoon, say, from 2.15 to 2.30. Settle down and worry about it. Give it your full attention and get as upset as you need to. No, honestly – try it. If you don't feel comfortable sitting down to it, do it while you're ironing. But only for 15 minutes – set a timer and stop when it buzzes. When you catch yourself worrying at other times, stop at once – but promise yourself you've only got to wait till 2.15.
- Wash it away. Worry to your heart's content while you're washing up or cleaning floors – but only then – and throw your worries out with the dirty water.
- Write it down. The whole dreadful story, and all the awful things that could happen. Then burn it or tear it into tiny pieces. The same when you're angry – write a steaming letter to the person who's upset you, then make sure you destroy it. Just don't send it!

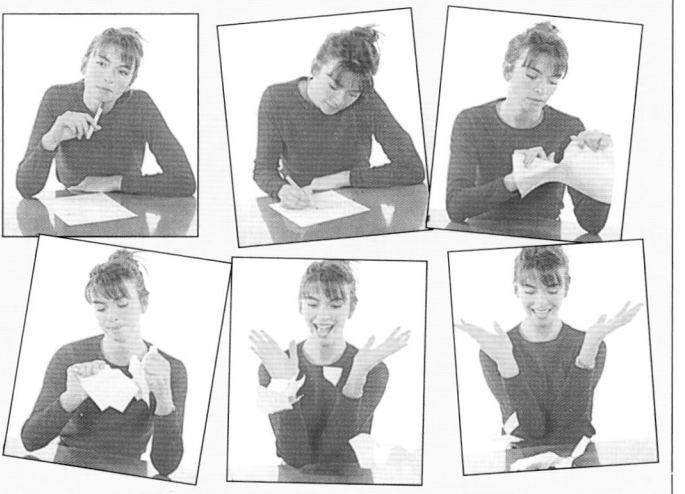

Hormonal Upheaval

No one can relax when they're suffering from premenstrual syndrome (PMS), which affects about three-quarters of us at one time or another. For most women it's a fairly mild nuisance – a bit of fluid retention making shoes and waistbands nip too tightly, a day or so when people seem unusually irritating or life looks bleak. Then their period starts and everything's back to normal. For some, though, it means major upheaval.

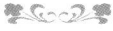

Wild moods, exhaustion, unbearable depression, tension, confusion, insomnia and thoughts of violence or suicide – PMS has even been used as a defence in murder trials.

Since PMS is caused by a temporary imbalance in the female hormones (too much oestrogen or too little progesterone) and possibly an imbalance in brain chemicals too, the answer is to try to balance things out again.

If all else fails, some gynaecologists now give hormone treatment. But self-help methods tackle the problem rather than the symptoms – and without drug side-effects.

◆ Keep moving. Energetic exercise makes the body produce feel-good chemicals called endorphins. Women are often low on these the week before a period, which accounts for the low spirits.

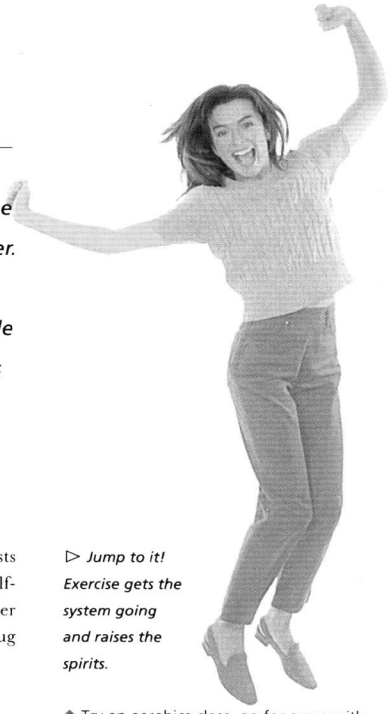

▷ *Jump to it! Exercise gets the system going and raises the spirits.*

◆ Try an aerobics class, go for a run with the dog or children, put on some lively music and dance all by yourself – anything to speed up your heart and get those endorphins moving.

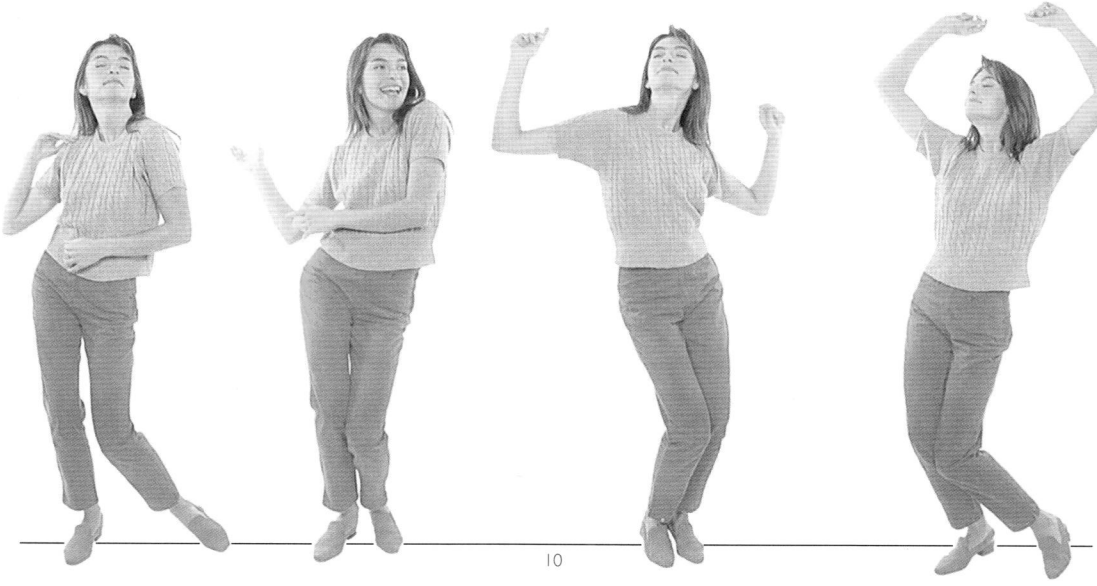

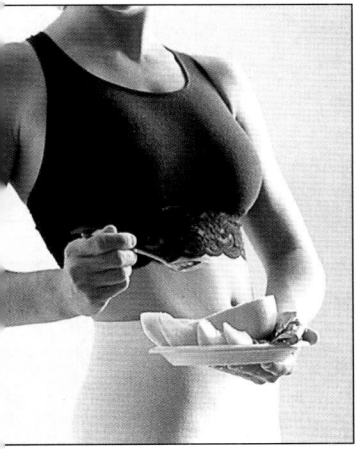

△ *Eat small healthy meals.*

◆ Eat little and often, especially if you find yourself wanting to nibble all the time. Instead of raiding the biscuit tin, have half a dozen small meals a day of wholesome carbohydrates like bread, pasta, fruit and vegetables. By keeping blood sugar levels steady, this helps prevent mood swings.

▽ *Put on some lively music and dance.*

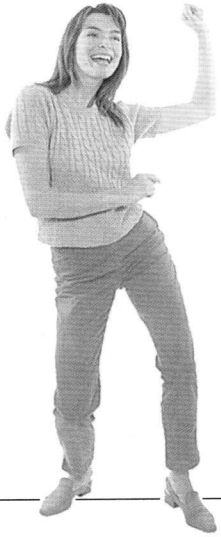

EAT TO BEAT THE BLUES

Changing your diet could solve PMS problems. Unfortunately, chocolate only cheers you up till you step on the scales – the solution is more likely to come in vegetable shape. Modern convenience food causes a lot of women's hormonal problems; it's packed with saturated fat, for instance, which makes the body produce too much oestrogen.

The Women's Nutritional Advisory Service (UK) finds that different kinds of PMS are caused, or made worse, by a shortage of nutrients. It provides tailor-made anti-PMS diets, including food supplements if necessary, but also offers some general advice:

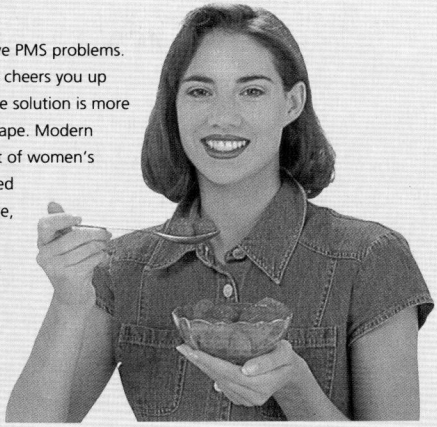

△ *A simple change of diet can work wonders.*

◆ For all forms of PMS, stock up on vitamin B6 and magnesium. If your symptoms tend to be nervous tension, mood swings and anxiety, these may be all you need. For more vitamin B6, eat fish, liver, bacon, beans, yeast extract, tomato puree and bananas. For magnesium, add muesli, oatmeal, dried fruit and dried skimmed milk. There's plenty of both in wholemeal bread, soya flour, mung beans and nuts.

◆ Weight gain, bloating and tender breasts, in addition to B6 and magnesium, add some vitamin E from oils (sunflower-seed, peanut, olive or cod-liver), nuts, salmon, tuna blackberries, spinach and avocado.

◆ Headaches, exhaustion, dizziness and craving for sweets; add chromium from rye bread, calf liver, eggs, brewer's yeast, peppers and potatoes.

◆ Depression, confusion and insomnia; you need vitamin C – weight for weight, there's even more in blackcurrants, parsley, canned guavas, strawberries, peppers and raw red cabbage than in oranges.

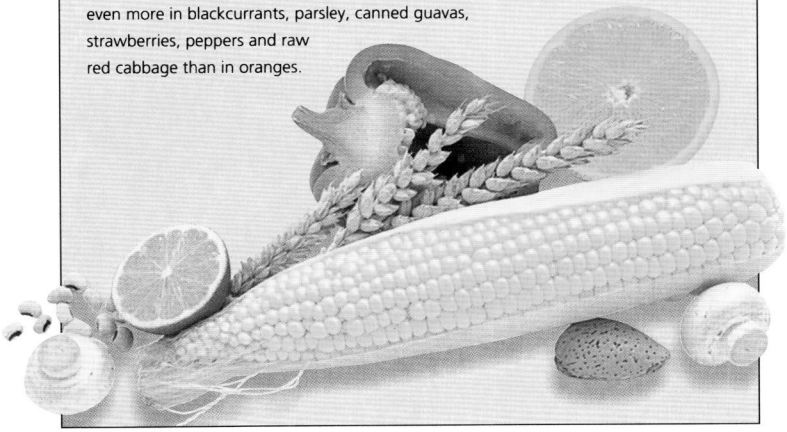

Peaceful Pregnancy

The image of a mother-to-be is a beautiful, tranquil creature drifting through soft-focus scenery, one hand on the neat little bump, the other stroking the head of a happy toddler. The reality, as most of us know or can guess, is rather different.

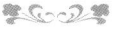

Today's mother-to-be is often either working until the last minute or caring for other children who aren't at all sensitive to her needs. The happy event may be overshadowed with financial worries or – especially if it's the first child – a secret fear that it might all be a terrible mistake.

Doubts and fears are perfectly natural. Having a child is, after all, a major change and a serious set of new responsibilities. Children restrict your freedom, make a mess, cost a fortune and never give you a day off. Bottling up these worries can cause a lot of unnecessary unhappiness, so talk it over with someone you trust.

Don't forget to welcome the new baby, though. It sounds bizarre, but many experts now believe the baby can sense your feelings about it. Unborn babies are certainly affected by their mother's moods, since these send hormones coursing through her bloodstream, which the baby shares. So when you're tense or angry the baby's going to be filled with the same stressful hormones.

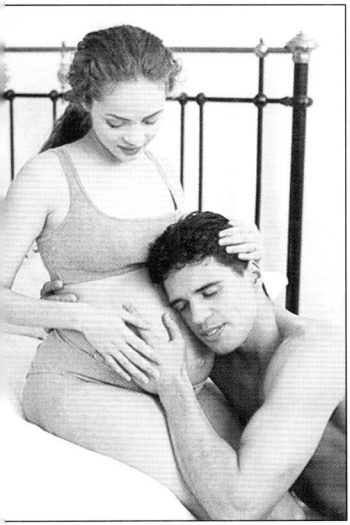

△ *Help the baby's father feel more involved.*

◁ *Give yourself time to relax each day.*

Also, the baby hears and responds to noises just as we do. Researchers have even discovered their taste in music – they don't like heavy metal, but relax to serene sounds like Mozart. Makes sense, really.

◆ Give yourself time to relax every day, using any of the methods in this book. Easier said than done, but well worth the effort if you take the phone off the hook and tell everyone you're doing this for your health.

◆ Help the baby's father feel involved by giving you backrubs – or even better, learning some massage techniques. Lie on your side with a pillow supporting your upper knee as you get bigger. Avoid pressure on the abdomen (especially in the first few months) and only use essential oils if they're guaranteed safe for use in pregnancy. Also let him rub your legs gently upwards from the ankles.

◆ If your doctor wants to give you iron tablets, ask for a blood test to see if you really need them. If you do, look for liquid versions that claim not to cause constipation.

◆ As well as giving up smoking, try not to let anyone smoke near you. On top of everything else, it raises the levels of stress hormones in the blood.

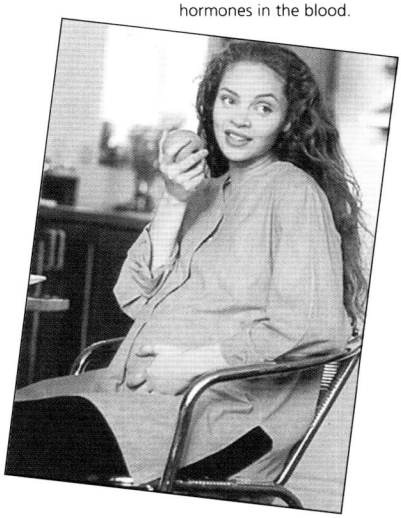

△ *A healthy balanced diet is very important.*

CAN YOU HEAR ME IN THERE?

Sit comfortably with hands on your abdomen, maybe in a rocking chair, and talk to the baby growing inside you. Say something like 'I'm looking forward to meeting you, and playing with you.' Tell it about the other members of the family, or what you've been doing that day. Just keep to positive subjects. You don't even have to talk out loud. What's happening is that you're encouraging your brain to produce calming, mood-lifting hormones. You'll feel good, and if the baby understands, all the better!

▷ *Tell the baby all about the other members of the family and introduce brothers and sisters at an early stage.*

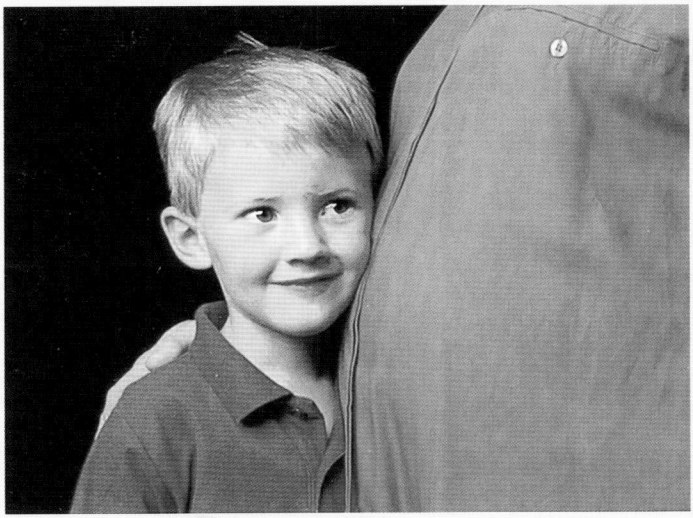

Relax? With Kids Like Mine?

Bringing up children, with all its rewards, gives women little chance to relax at the best of times. Looking after hyperactive children makes it virtually impossible.

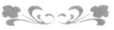

Sometimes bad behaviour is caused by emotional problems which call for counselling, preferably on referral from a doctor. Homeopathy can also be useful. Sometimes kids just need a grown-up to spend time listening to them. And of course, if they see adults being angry they learn to do the same. Local parents' groups can be helpful when you're feeling isolated and under pressure.

With many children, though, one look at their flushed faces and glazed eyes shows it's out of their control. They look as if they've been drugged, and in a sense they have. What with air pollution, passive smoking and the use of chemicals in the food industry, their small bodies can get a toxic overload.

Healthy eating helps children fight off the effects of traffic fumes and other pollutants. If you live in an old house with lead pipes in a soft-water area, let the tap run fast for half a minute before using the water first thing in the morning.

Some children are more sensitive than others to the over-stimulating effects of nicotine, so try not to let anyone smoke indoors, where fumes don't have a chance to disperse.

Many parents find the problem is caused by food additives. Once you know what foods contain a particular additive the connection may become obvious, when the child starts acting up straight after eating or drinking it. Occasionally a child is allergic to some normally wholesome food. If you suspect this, see an allergy consultant or ask your doctor to refer you to a dietician.

A surprising number of children simply don't eat enough – it's exhaustion that makes them so bad-tempered. Children who miss breakfast, in particular, get into more trouble at school and have lower exam results than those who start the day with a meal. Snacking on junk food just makes matters worse, because it's full of things – like the caffeine in cola drinks and chocolate – that can make them moody and restless. Picky eaters are maddening, but perseverance pays off for everyone.

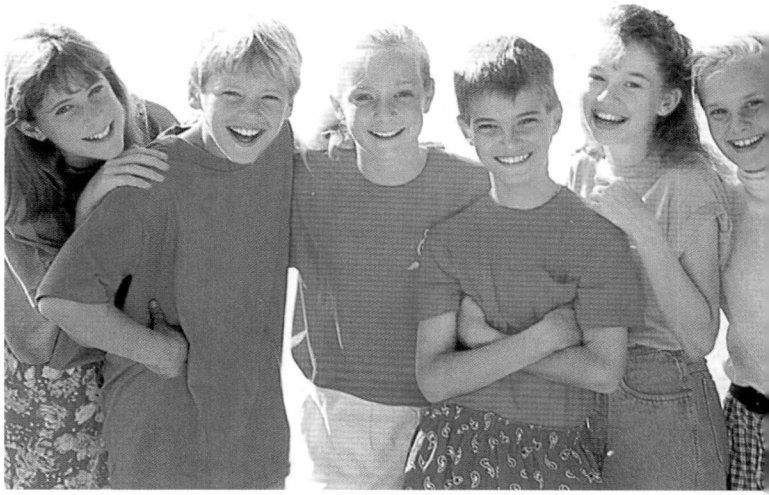

△ *Children who eat a balanced and varied diet, snacking on fruit rather than junk food, will be full of vitality.*

BAD GUYS OR BAD GRUB?

Several American prisons have reduced violence by giving inmates a healthier diet containing more magnesium, selenium and chromium and less sugar.

◆ So try feeding your own tearaways on wholemeal bread, Marmit (brewer's yeast), leafy green vegetables, beans, onions, apricots, bananas and grapes.

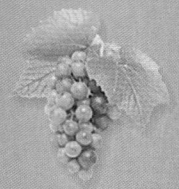

◆ Don't give vitamin or mineral supplements except in special formulations for children.

◁ *Fresh air, fresh food, unpolluted air and water are vital to the whole family's health.*

SOOTHING A WILD CHILD

◆ Adding a few drops of calming aromatherapy oil like camomile or benzoin to a child's bath, mixed with a carrier oil for safety, can aid a good night's sleep. A small child may accept being massaged with it. During the day, use it in an oil burner.

◆ Blue and green are calming colours for clothes and bedrooms. A hop pillow will help restless children sleep.

◆ Herbal teas – not heavily sugared herbal toddler drinks – can be soothing, if the child will drink them.

◆ Herbalist Penelope Ody recommends a weak 'tea' made with 10g of the herbs agrimony and self-heal in a mug of hot water, sweetened with honey.

◆ With herbs and oils, use quarter-strength for small children, half-strength when they're older. Don't let them put essential oils, even blended, in their mouths.

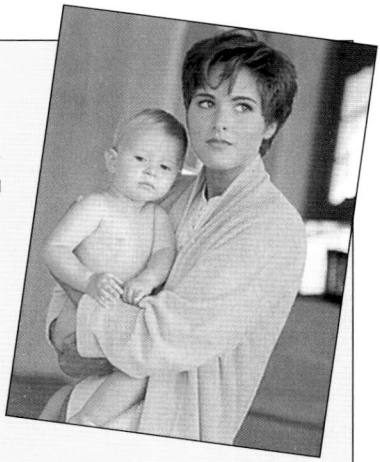

△ *Food allergies or deficiencies may cause a child to be restless.*

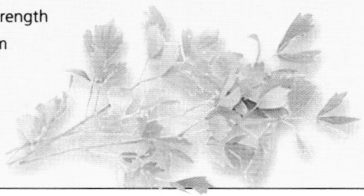

Moving With The Change

Until recently, menopause was seen as a dreary time of health problems and endings. Now, luckily, women look at life more positively. There's no longer any need to define ourselves by our youth or ability to have children. Most of us will be working for at least another decade. Our activities, families and friends are there to help us through low times.

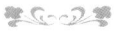

The menopause is another of life's transitions, like your first day at school, puberty, setting up home and having children. Not all the changes are necessarily welcome. But this can be one of the most energetic times of a woman's life. Even old age needn't be frightening if you plan for it and look after your health.

◆ Take some energetic exercise at least three times a week, to keep depression – and weight-gain – at bay. If it's also weight-bearing exercise (say aerobics or running) you'll be keeping your bones strong too. This reduces your risk of the brittle-bone disease osteoporosis, one of the major problems faced by older women.

◆ When you feel stressed and irritable, find a quiet spot to do your favourite relaxation technique, take a walk or watch a cartoon video. Organize for your own needs instead of everyone else's.

▽ ***We need not be afraid of growing older if we keep a positive outlook.***

SAYING GOODBYE

It's no use pretending losses aren't painful. Sometimes a letting-go ritual can help you say goodbye and move on.

Write a letter to the person or thing you've lost, whether it's your job, your marriage, your children who've left home, or anything else. Be clear what you're missing. If you're mourning your youth, for example, is it your fertility, your role as mother, your youthful looks? Or all of these? Do you suspect your sex life is over? Do you think you'll be despised and ignored? Do you fear weakness and ill-health?

Write it down without holding anything back. When you've got it all out, spend some time thinking it over and let yourself cry as much as you want. Then burn the letter and blow the ashes out of the window. Take a few deep breaths and say 'I'm moving on to the rest of my life'. Then do something you enjoy, preferably with friends.

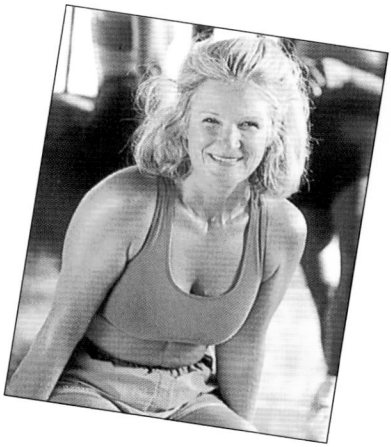

△ *Regular energetic exercise will help to keep bones strong.*

◆ Hormone replacement therapy helps some women, but find out about all the options. The Women's Nutritional Advisory Service offers natural alternatives.

◆ Cut down on animal fats, coffee, fizzy drinks, sugar and alcohol but eat plenty of fresh vegetables and fruit. This will protect your bones as well as helping keep your moods on an even keel. Japanese women, who rarely suffer menopausal symptoms, eat masses of vegetables and soya products such as tofu (beancurd).

◆ The advice for PMS (page 10) is helpful for menopausal problems too.

◆ Make time to go out with friends. If they've melted away over the years, find some more through evening classes or community groups. Talk problems over when you need to, but don't get into downbeat habits. Spend time with people who buck you up instead of bringing you down.

◆ Promise yourself at least one thing a week that's nothing but fun. Look through the local paper for new things to do and book ahead.

△ *Our activities, families and friends are there to help us when we need a little help.*

◁ *Make time to see friends regularly. Enjoy yourself and have fun.*

Coping With Pain

It's hard to relax when you're in pain, but that's when it does most good. Pain and tension fuel each other in a vicious cycle of distress. Relaxation is especially vital in conditions like backache when muscles go into spasm around the painful spot – that's meant to protect the area from further damage, but its main effect is to hurt even more.

Illness is a powerful source of anxiety, and sometimes the treatments seem as disruptive as the disease. Though it's difficult to keep your mind on learning new techniques, this is a good time to take up relaxation. As well as speeding recovery, it could help prevent relapses.

◆ Try foot-to-head relaxation, meditation, visualising yourself free of pain, plus any other techniques your doctor thinks suitable.
◆ Have you taken all practical steps to combat whatever's causing the pain?
◆ Go to your doctor if you have any unexplained pain – and get a second opinion if the first isn't helpful.

Mind over matter

Can you outwit pain or imagine it away? When nothing else is working or you don't want to fill yourself with painkillers, it's worth a try. It may take a while, but these methods have worked for many people. Lie or sit in any position you find comfortable and give yourself time. Starting with some breathing exercises or meditation may help.

◆ Imagine a ray of light warming and healing the painful spot. Really feel the warmth and the comfort.

◆ See your pain as a wild animal, snarling and ferocious. Approach it safely – you're in control – then stroke it and soothe it till it calms down.

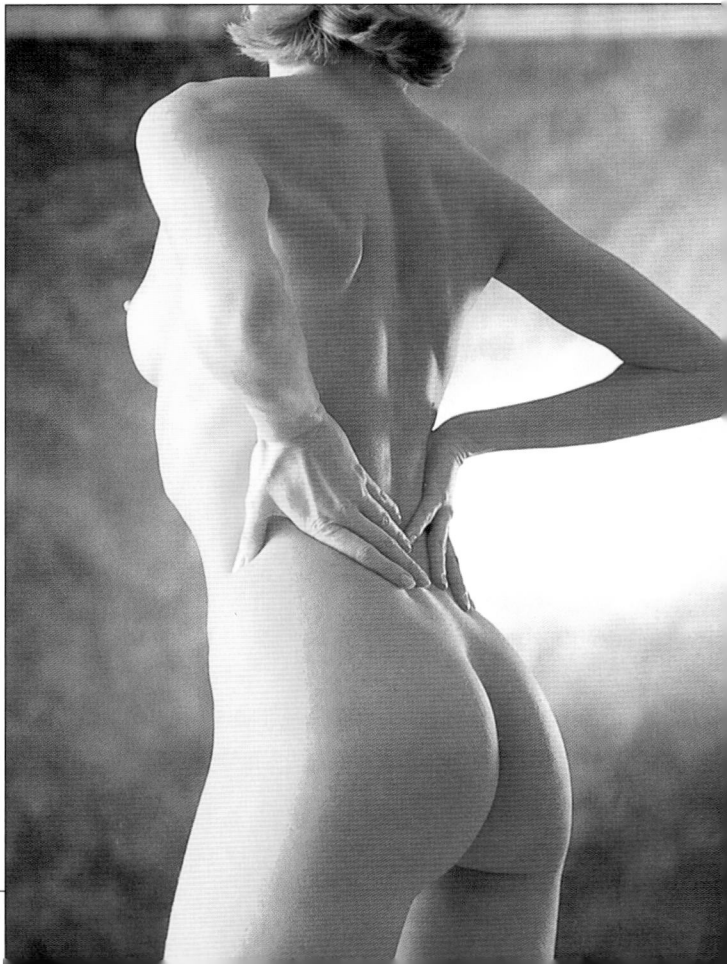

▽ *Back pain is common, but luckily there's a lot you can do to relieve it, especially by improving the way you stand and sit.*

BE KIND TO YOUR BACK

Most women suffer backache at some time in their lives, what with periods, pregnancy, office work, high heels, carrying toddlers or just being on their feet all day.

- A rucksack distributes weight more evenly than handbags or shoulder bags.
- For the same reason, use a baby sling or backpack-style carrier instead of toting Junior on your hip.
- If your bed's soft or more than 10 years old you may be sagging while you sleep. Treat yourself to a firm new mattress.
- Make sure your work equipment – kitchen surfaces, office furniture – is the right height.
- Improve your posture, say with the Alexander Technique. Especially, tuck your tail under so the forward curve at your waist is slightly flattened. An exaggerated curve looks elegant but wrecks your spine.
- Bend your knees, not your back, to pick things up (see picture sequence, right).
- Unless your doctor insists, staying active helps a bad back more than resting.
- Avoid any exercise that includes tipping your head backwards, straight-legged toe-touching or 'windmilling', lifting both legs together or violent twists.
- Yoga, stretching and aerobic exercise can ease period-related backache.
- Ask your doctor if there's a local back-care clinic for more advice and special exercises.

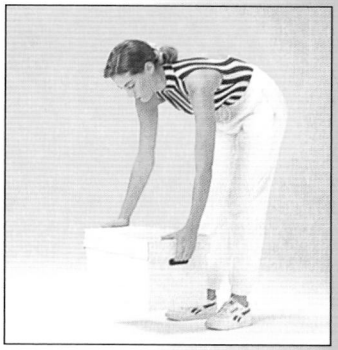

△ *Lifting like this can cause back problems.*

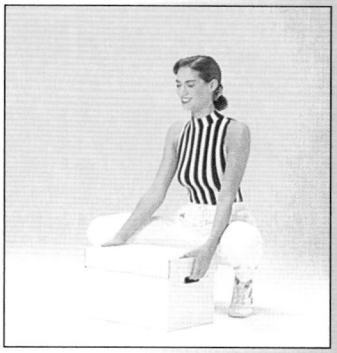

△ *Bend your knees, lifting with back straight.*

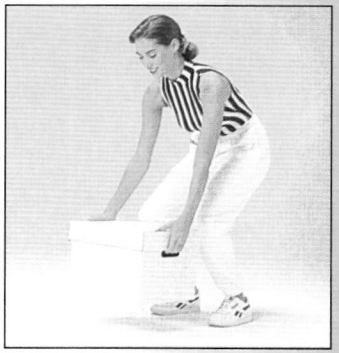

△ *Put things down with a straight spine, too.*

- Imagine the pain as something you can see – a rock, a blade, a blob of colour – and fix your attention on it. How big is it? What colour? What shape? Does it have a sound? A smell? Is it moving? The images will keep changing, but eventually you may wear it out. And by facing the pain you lose the fear that makes your muscles knot up so painfully.

◁ *When you don't want to reach for the painkillers, it may be worth trying to imagine the pain away. Meditation or breathing exercises may help.*

Stress Relief First Aid

Many of the techniques in this book are quick and effective. Breathing exercises don't have to take more than a minute, and five minutes is enough to meditate or do a short foot-to-head muscle relaxation. While you're reading this book, why not put an 'x' in the margin beside your favourite quick relaxers so you can find them when you need them fast?

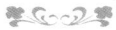

When everything's getting on top of you, give yourself a break. That old advice about taking a deep breath still holds good – count to 10 as you breathe out. If you're paralysed with anxiety, do a breathing exercise and clear your mind by concentrating on the feel of your breath. Start by blowing out hard to empty your lungs and let a deep breath in. If you feel faint, lie down with your feet higher than your head. If you feel like hitting someone, go for a walk instead.

Taking your mind off the problem can help – things are easier to cope with when you're not at the peak of stress. So read a light magazine feature or the stars (but only believe them if they're good). Make a cup of herbal tea and ring your best friend for some moral support. If you can't get the worry off your mind, put your brain to work recalling one of Shakespeare's sonnets, or counting backwards in threes from 100.

Meanwhile, here are some extra emergency tips.

Five seconds to spare

Just enough time for some encouraging affirmations – positive messages to the subconscious to boost your confidence. Silently tell yourself 'I'm doing well' and 'I can easily cope with all of this'. Never mind if you don't believe it – say it as if you do. Repeat it a few times whenever you think of it. And if any mean inner voices start quibbling, imagine them coming from a radio and turn it off.

Ten seconds to spare

Stand straight and breathe in through your nose as you stretch your arms above your head, palms together.

As you start breathing out through your mouth, turn the palms out and slowly bring the arms down beside you, reaching out with the fingertips. As your arms come down, tell yourself 'I am perfectly calm'.

If people are around, just pinch the web between your thumb and first finger (don't do this if you're pregnant) and breathe deeply.

Twenty seconds to spare

With feet apart, breathe in deeply while you stand on your toes and clench all your muscles. Breathing out slowly while you sink to the floor, let everything relax.

Don't get extra stressed if you can't balance on your toes, just do all the rest.

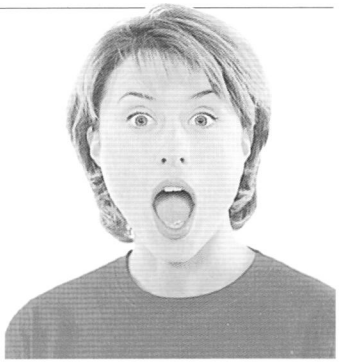

Half a minute to spare

Scrunch your face into a wicked scowl, relax with your mouth hanging open, repeat this two or three times, then put on a smile even if you don't feel like it. Massage your scalp in little circles with the pads of your fingers. Relaxing the face and scalp keeps tension headaches at bay while the very movement of smiling sends calming signals to the brain.

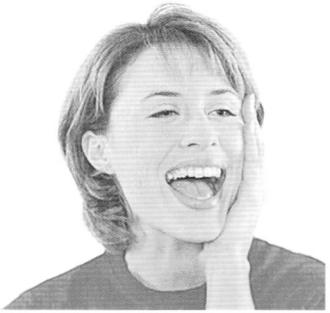

One minute stress relief

Laughter is a great stress-reliever – scan the cartoons in the newspaper or phone a telephone jokeline. Keep a book by your favourite funny person for when you're feeling desperate, and reread the parts that made you laugh most.

Ten second stress relief first aid

▷ *Stand straight, breathe through your nose as you stretch your arms above your head, palms together.*

▷ *Start breathing out through your mouth, turn palms out and slowly bring your arms down to your sides.*

▷ *Reaching out with your finger-tips, as your arms come down, tell yourself 'I am perfectly calm'.*

Twenty second stress relief first aid

◁ *With feet apart, breathe in deeply. Stand on your toes and clench all your muscles.*

◁ *Breathe out slowly while you sink to the floor.*

◁ *Let everything relax.*

Half a minute to spare

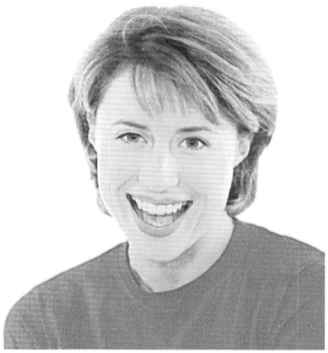

△ *Put on a smile even if you don't feel like it.*

Eat to Stay on Top

Anyone who's felt jumpy after too many coffees, or struggled to solve simple work problems after missing breakfast, knows that food affects our state of mind as well as our physical health.

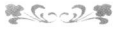

Under stress, eating well is more important than ever. Vegetables, wholemeal bread, beans, dairy products and eggs, for example, provide plentiful B vitamins to build strong nerves. Stress also wears down the immune system, which is why we fall ill at difficult times – all the more reason to eat healthy food that boosts our defences.

We thrive on simple, natural foods, a wide variety of fresh vegetables, fruit, whole grains (brown bread, rice, pasta and cereals), some protein (fish, meat, dairy or vegetarian products like tofu) and some olive or vegetable oil.

You don't have to leave out all your old treats, as long as most of what you're eating comes from this healthy list. Things like bread, pasta, fruit and vegetables – complex carbohydrates – are very filling but not fattening if you don't pile on rich sauces and spreads.

Modern processed foods, on the other hand, tend to be unhealthily packed with sugar, salt, white flour, saturated fat and artificial additives. They take the place of the nutrient-rich foods we need, and can even deplete our supplies of vitamins and minerals in trying to digest them.

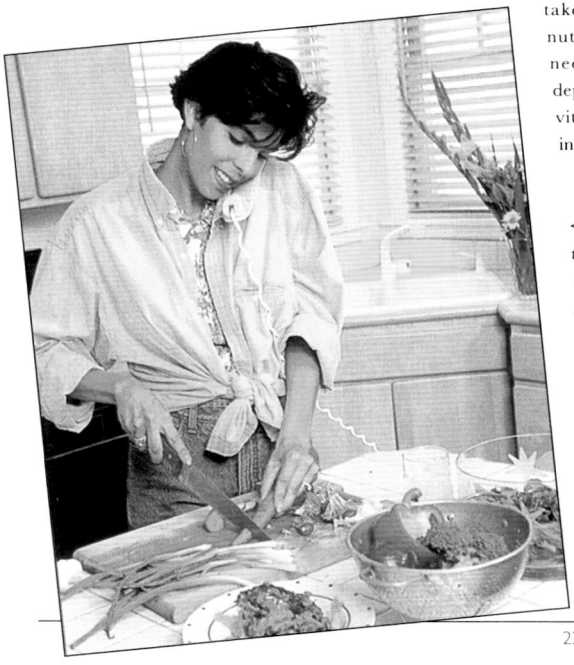

◁ The less processed the food you eat, the more it will do for you. Fresh fruit and vegetables are top of the list.

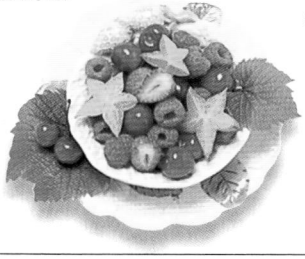

A heavy meal leaves you feeling sleepy, while a high-protein supper can keep you awake. Rich foods can make you lethargic, while caffeine (in chocolate as well as tea and coffee) gives you the jitters.

Too much sugar or salt may disrupt the body's chemical and mineral balance, causing mood swings among other harmful effects. Missing a meal, especially breakfast, makes blood sugar levels fall so low that the brain can't function properly – you feel irritable and may have more accidents.

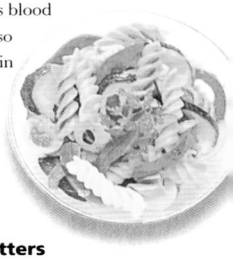

Weighty matters

If you overeat for comfort, swap to healthier treats such as fresh fruit – try a mango, a banana and a handful of cherries. Have some chocolate or chips if you want them but eat slowly, savouring the taste. Stop when you've had enough, knowing you can eat them whenever you really want to (forbidden fruit is so much more tempting). And you don't have to clear your plate or finish unwanted leftovers. Throw them to the birds.

Beware of not eating enough, though. Most slimming diets lack essential nutrients and keep blood sugar levels low. Dieters gain poorer scores in intelligence tests. Fortunately, the best diet for long-term weight-loss is also the best for vibrant health and serenity – low in fat, high in fresh vegetables and unprocessed foods.

ENERGY FOODS

- Inadequate carbohydrate intake can result in fatigue and poor energy levels.
- Pasta, rice, cereals, bread, fruit and potatoes are a good source of carbohydrate energy.

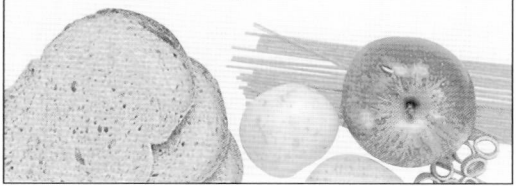

SUPER STRESS-BUSTERS

- Bananas
- Mackerel
- Marmite (brewer's yeast)
- Chillis
- Citrus fruit
- Wholemeal bread
- Oats
- Brazil nuts
- Lettuce
- Leafy green vegetables

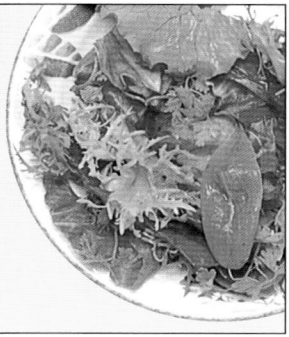

SPEED TRAPS

Take a short break while you eat, even if it's only 10 minutes, making time to chew your food properly and enjoy it. Eating in a rush can trigger the release of stress hormones as well as causing indigestion.

For a healthy snack, nibble some nuts and raisins, fresh fruit, wholemeal sandwiches with salad or a bowl of good breakfast cereal like Weetabix, Corn Flakes or low-sugar muesli.

Organize to Avoid Stress

This is for everyone who says 'I haven't got time to relax'. One of the best pieces of advice I've ever read was in a women's magazine years ago. It said, 'If you never put things down but always put them away, you'll never have to tidy up again.' How true that is – and it comes back to haunt me every time I'm 'too busy' to put things away as I go along.

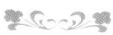

Fast food seems handy when you're too busy to prepare fresh vegetables and eat properly. But as your energy levels sink and you start catching endless infections you lose all the time you gained, and more besides.

Being organized is the best way of making extra time in your life and cutting down stress. Admittedly, anyone with children, a home and a job may feel she's doing all the organizing a human being can possibly do. Yet there's frequently room to make things easier for ourselves. When you've done things in a certain way for years, you can sometimes get a blind spot about doing them any other way.

If you know someone who seems to be less overworked (and not because she married a millionaire) why not ask how she does it? Share tips with your friends, you will all have different ideas. Think what a wealth of experience you've got, so have other people, and you may be able to use it. Professional organizer Denise Katz has five golden rules:

- Do it now
- Be prepared
- Work at your own pace
- Don't aim for perfection
- Sort out your priorities.

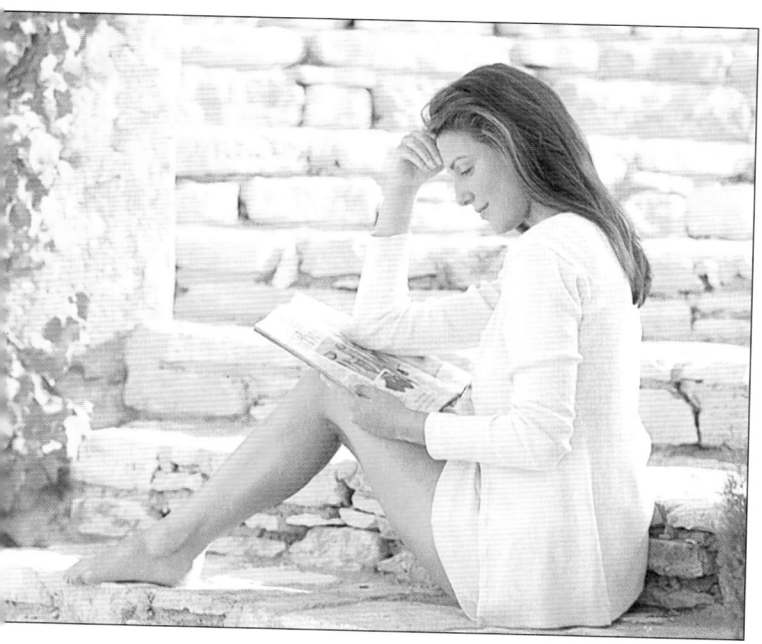

Time to reorganize

One thing I'm not suggesting is that you reorganize your day to find time for a dozen more things. If it's already hectic, which is why you're reading a book on stress relief, please don't add any extra commitments. It's better to look at all the things you're already doing and ask if you could leave any of them out.

If you don't work for the pure love of it, could you afford to work shorter hours, and use the extra time more enjoyably doing cheaper things? Could you join a bartering scheme, for example, or perhaps grow some of your own food?

Ask yourself if anything you're doing will seem like a waste of time when you look back on it in a year. And above all, don't feel guilty.

◁ Everyone needs time to relax and recover from the stresses of the day. So don't feel bad about spending time on yourself.

TIME FOR YOU

Schedule a time for relaxation, even if it's only 15 minutes after the children are in bed and before you start clearing up.

◆ Promise yourself (and tell everyone) you're not going to think of anyone else in the time you have set yourself.

◆ Setting a timer will save you worrying you'll fall asleep. Have a quick check that nothing catastrophic is likely to happen – more to stop you leaping up with a cry of 'Have I left the gas on?' than anything else – then unplug the phone and begin.

◆ Swap childcare/relaxation time with a friend. Or practice some of the techniques together – as with exercise, friends can encourage each other.

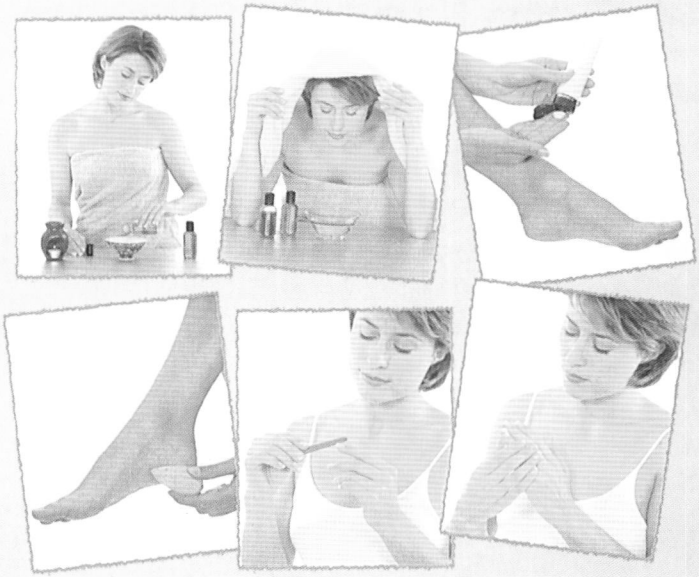

▷ *Make time to pamper yourself.*

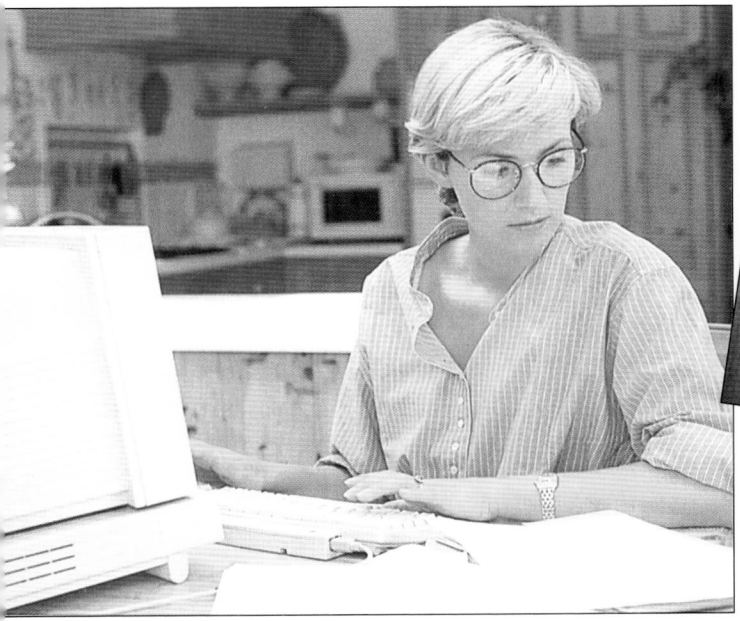

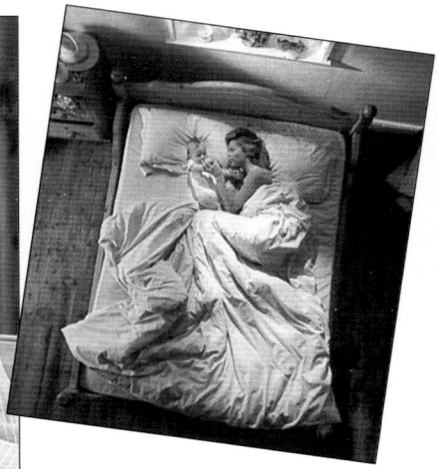

△ *Spend some time doing the things you want to do and then return refreshed and revived to deal with the demands of the day.*

◁ *Put your skills to work so you can reorganize your routine to save valuable time.*

A Safe Place to Relax

Ideally, we'd all have a room we could lock ourselves away in whenever we needed some time to ourselves. An uncluttered spot that's used for nothing else, so it always has a peaceful atmosphere. Small is fine – determined relaxers have emptied boxrooms, taken over a second bathroom or put an oil heater in the shed.

For most of us, it's a question of finding a quiet spot to call our own. A corner of the bedroom is the likeliest place, as privacy is important – you won't want an audience for your face or voice exercises. Make sure everyone knows it's your place to relax – they're not to interrupt you while you're there or pile washing on your chair when you're not.

Try to find a spot that's not associated with any other activity. You want to establish this as the place where you relax. We are creatures of habit so, once you've used this place several times, you'll find you start to relax as soon as you sit down there. Here's what you need:

- A wooden chair, unless you're very used to sitting straight-backed on the floor – as in yoga.
- Space to stretch out on your back.

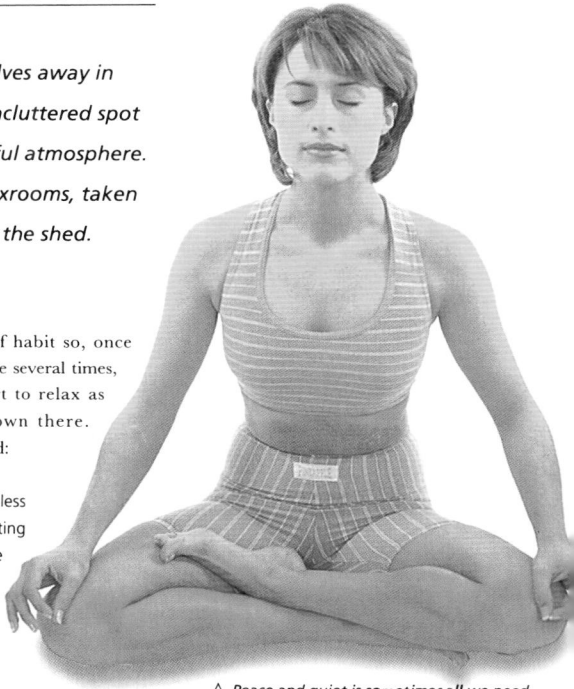

△ *Peace and quiet is sometimes all we need.*

- A table, mantelpiece or bookshelf to burn candles and keep any other equipment on.
- A pile of candles, a candlestick and a box of matches.
- An oil burner and a few of your favourite scented oils.
- A cassette player and relaxing music or meditation tapes.
- Surroundings as uncluttered as possible.
- A picture of peaceful scenery, such as woodland or the sea. Instead of displaying it permanently, you could also make putting up your poster part of your relaxation ritual.

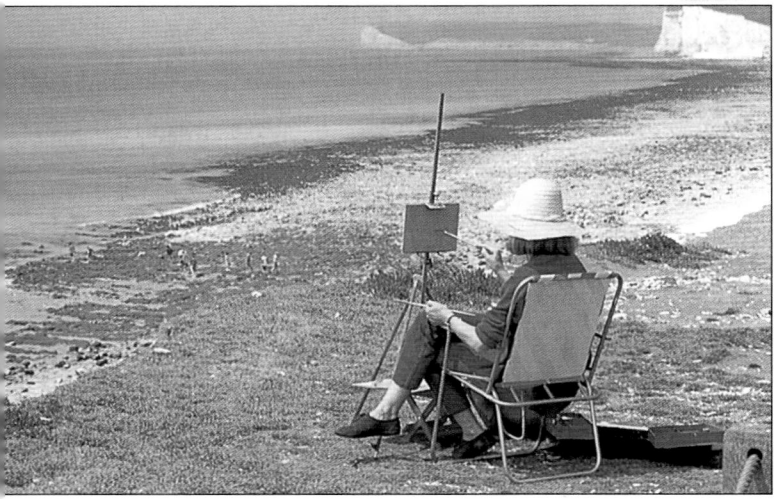

◁ *Your own safe place to relax may be real or imaginary.*

YOUR INNER REFUGE

My relaxation room is painted in pale colours with a big window, filmy curtains, deep carpet, a tranquil painting on the wall and a few inspiring objects; statues, crystals and candles. There's a small indoor fountain too, and a Persian rug to lie on. Though it's upstairs, overlooking wooded hills, I can step out whenever I like into a well kept garden where roses bloom all year. Needless to say it's rent-free and never needs dusting, since it exists only in my head.

Whatever the limitations on our physical space, this is the sort of place we can all have – an inner refuge. When I close my eyes to relax I can be sitting in this peaceful room, or in dappled light under a tree, or on a riverbank or sea shore. Daydreaming? No, using a time-honoured method of restoring my mental health in a hectic day.

◆ Imagine a room or outdoor scene where you feel perfectly at peace. Use a picture from a magazine or make it up yourself, but visualize all the details. What's the pattern on the curtains? What flowers are there? How does the grass feel under your feet? When you're tired and stressed, imagine yourself resting there.

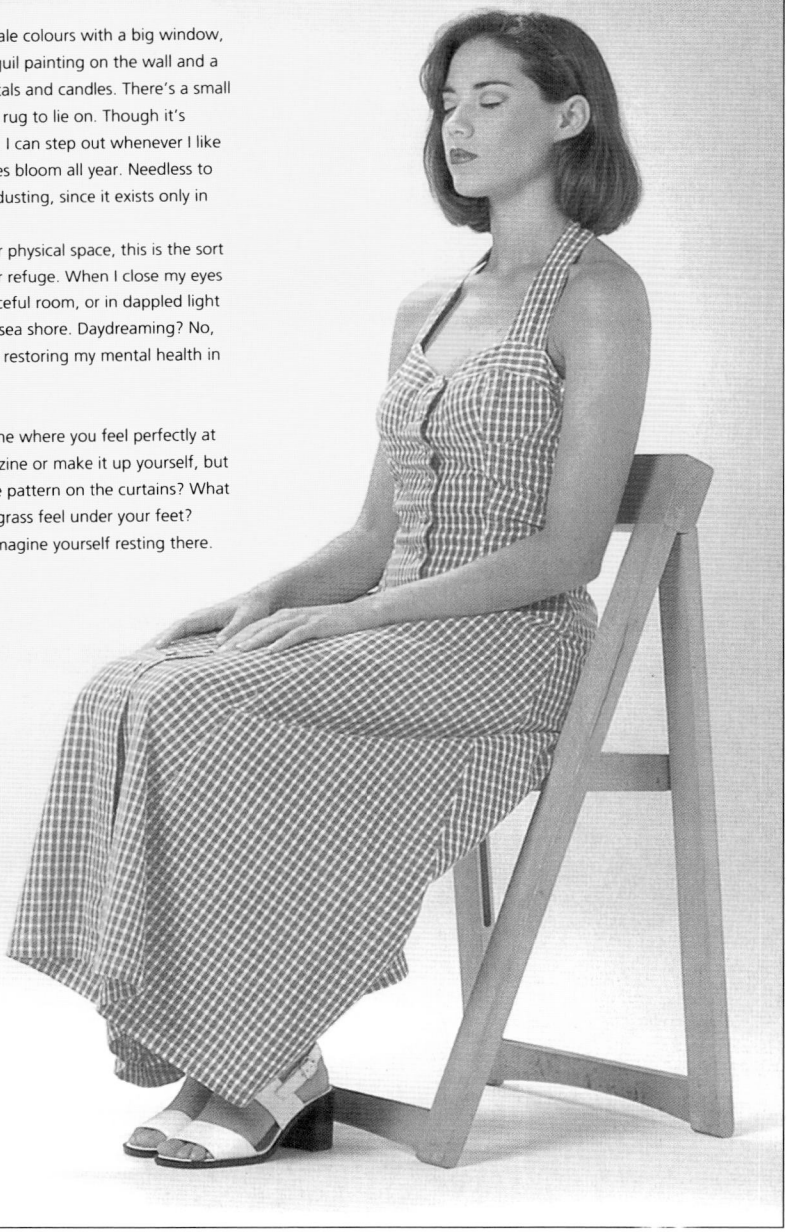

Breathe Your Troubles Away

One of the simplest ways of relieving tension is by breathing well – which most of us don't do. Put one hand on your chest and the other on your navel – if the lower hand doesn't move, you're not breathing deeply enough. Forget about flattening your stomach and let in a good deep breath.

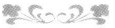

While shallow breathing produces the stress hormone adrenaline, a deep breath puts masses of oxygen into the bloodstream for an instant health boost to the whole body. No wonder it clears our heads, it's feeding our brains. Simply learning to breathe fully is a powerful way of relieving stress. Keep checking during the day till you do it constantly, not too deeply, but in a natural rhythm.

◆ Don't overdo the oxygen – you can have too much of a good thing. If you're feeling light-headed, either from breathing too deeply or from gulping in air under stress, breathe in and out of a paper bag a few times to restore the balance of oxygen and carbon dioxide.

◆ Check with your doctor before doing breathing exercises if you have epilepsy or high blood pressure.

Breathing fully

Find a quiet spot to sit comfortably, with your back straight. It doesn't matter if you sit cross-legged, with or without your back resting against the wall, or on a straight-backed chair with feet flat on the floor.

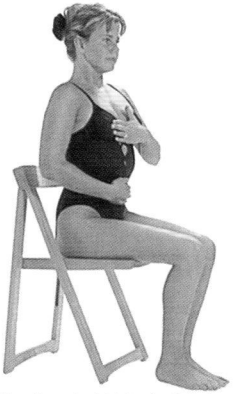

△ *Sitting in a straight-backed chair, put one hand on your tummy and the other on your chest as you breathe in through your nose.*

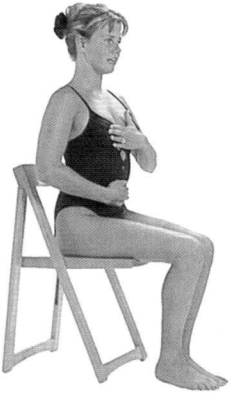

△ *As you breathe out through your mouth you will feel your chest and tummy move as the air is expelled.*

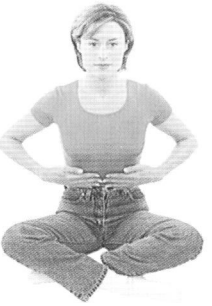

△ *As you take a deep breath through your nose, feel the abdomen rise and see the movement parting your fingertips.*

◆ If you're breathing fast, give yourself a minute to let it slow down naturally. Then put your hands side by side on your abdomen, fingertips meeting at or just below the navel.

◆ Take a deep breath through your nose and feel the oxygen pouring into every corner of your lungs. Feel the abdomen rise and watch the movement parting your fingertips. Breathe out and do it again, this time feeling your chest expand as well. Stop taking deep breaths and let your natural rhythm establish itself.

◆ Don't worry if it's not happening. If you're very used to holding your tummy in, you may need to push it out deliberately. The very act of making space there will let more air in.

LOVE BREATHING

Breathing deeply and calmly, say silently to yourself 'I breathe in peace' on the inbreath and 'I breathe out love' on the outbreath. If you're worried about someone, imagine this protective cloud of love enveloping them.

HA BREATHING

◆ Breathe in deeply through your nose, bringing your shoulders back to open your chest.

◆ Breathe out through your mouth with a long 'hhhhh' or 'haaaa' noise like a deep sigh, letting your shoulders relax and drop down. Try to make the outbreath longer than the inbreath.

◆ Repeat two or three times.

◆ Finish by relaxing for a moment with your eyes shut as you let your normal breathing pattern return.

◆ A variation of this works wonders if you're feeling so tense that you can't stop holding your breath. Simply puff all your breath out as far and as fast as you can, with a sharp 'ha!'. Then let a fresh breath in slowly to fill the space.

SINGLE-NOSTRIL BREATHING

◆ Breathe through one nostril at a time, keeping the other one covered.

◆ Breathe fully but not unnaturally slowly or deeply.

◆ After about a minute change to the other nostril.

◆ If you find this exercise difficult, try Ha Breathing.

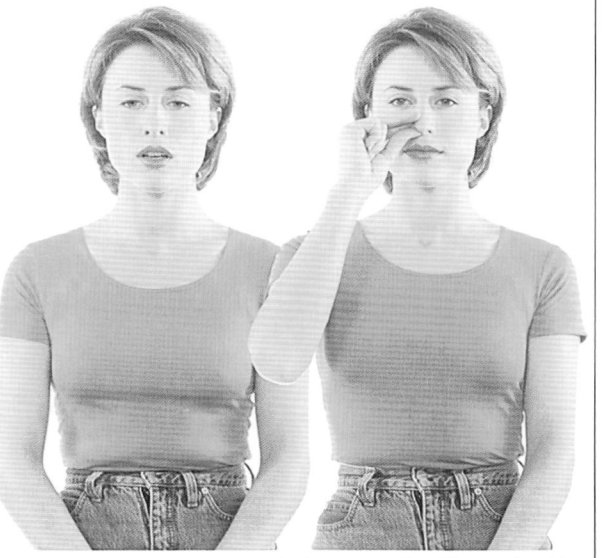

△ *Relax after Ha Breathing.* △ *Close one nostril and focus on breathing.*

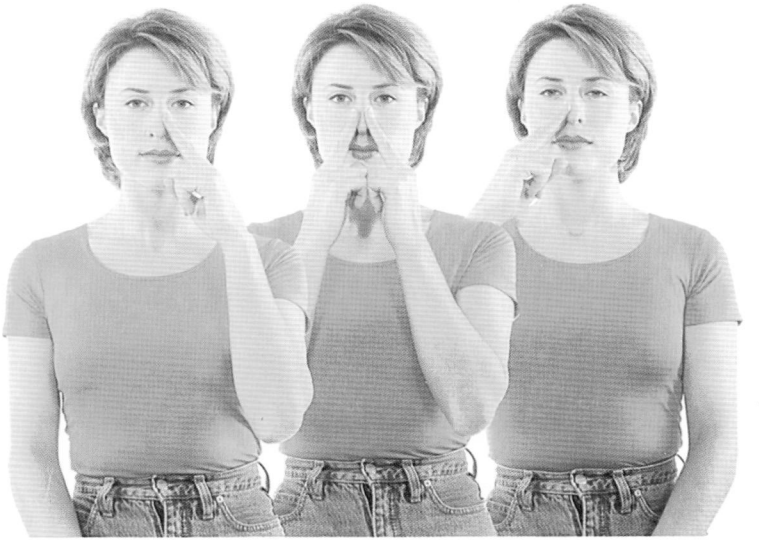

ALTERNATE NOSTRIL BREATHING

◆ Cover your left nostril with one finger and breathe in through the right while you count four seconds.

◆ Close both nostrils and count to two while you hold your breath. (Leave out this step if you have high blood pressure).

◆ Uncover your left nostril and breathe out to the count of four.

◆ Keep both nostrils closed for two seconds with your lungs empty.

◆ Uncover your left nostril again and breathe in through it while you count four seconds again.

◆ Close both nostrils for two seconds.

◆ Cover left nostril and breathe out through the right for four seconds.

◆ Repeat this whole cycle three more times.

Taking It From The Top

One of the first places stress makes itself felt is in our necks and shoulders. The face and spine also carry more than their share. How many times have you gritted your teeth, felt the weight of the world on your shoulders or found something a pain in the neck? People didn't pull those expressions out of the air – they're what really happens.

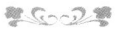

When a moment of stress passes we rarely leap or roll on the floor with joy, letting the tension out again. It just stays and builds up, contributing to migraine, repetitive strain injury, toothache and back pain.

Try a few easy exercises, particularly good for office workers or anyone who spends a lot of time sitting and using their hands. You can do them sitting down, but all the better if you can seize the chance to get up and move around a bit. Repeat all except the first and the last two exercises five times.

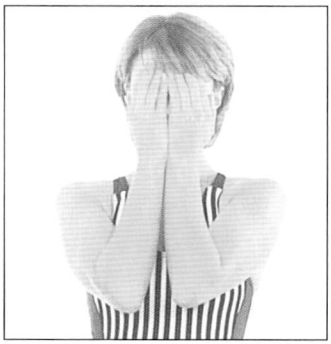

△ *Cup your hands over your eyes for a minute.*

- Rub your hands together to warm them, then cup them over your eyes for a minute.
- Lift your shoulders to your ears, keep them there for a moment, then let them drop. (Be careful to look ahead as you do this or you could get a horrible crick in the neck.)
- Look slowly from side to side, turning your head to look over your left shoulder and then your right.
- Let your head fall gently forward, bringing your chin as near your chest as possible. Slowly swing it in a U-shape, bringing your chin to your left shoulder, down again and to the right. Be careful not to go further than the shoulder or let your head tip directly backwards.
- Stretch your arms as high above your head as you can reach.
- With arms hanging down, lift your shoulders up, backwards and continuing in a circle.
- Stretch your arms out in front of you like a sleep walker, clench your fists, then quickly open them, stretching your fingers out. Flash them open and shut 10 times.
- Standing up, give your hair a good shake for a few seconds. Shake your hands, then your arms and finally each leg. Run on the spot, shaking your arms till you've shaken all the knots out.

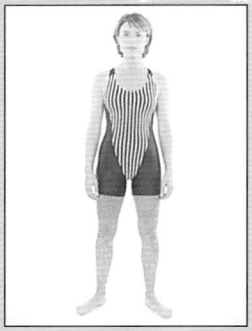

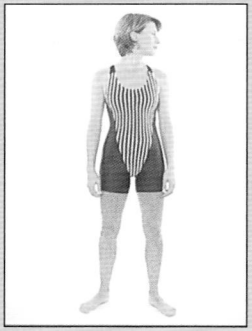

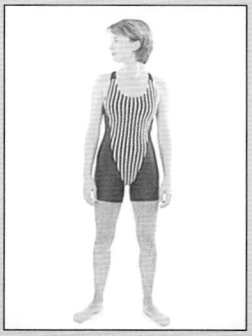

△ *Look slowly from side to side, turning your head to look over each shoulder in turn.*

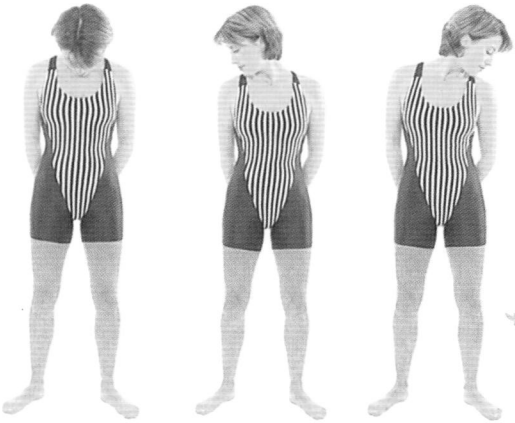

▷ *Let your head fall gently forward and slowly swing it in a U-shape, bringing your chin to each shoulder in turn.*

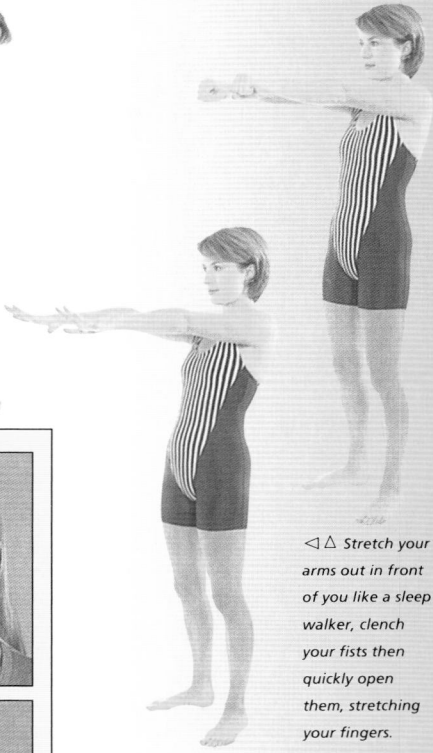

◁ △ *Stretch your arms out in front of you like a sleep walker, clench your fists then quickly open them, stretching your fingers.*

FUNNY FACE

Nobody looking? Give your face a much needed treat – it holds a lot of tension too.

◆ Open your eyes and mouth as wide as they'll go. Stick your tongue out and try to touch your nose.

◆ Purse your lips and push them forward, then stretch your mouth into a grin.

◆ Roll your eyes a few times. Raise your eyebrows into your hairline, then bring them down as far as you can and grimace.

◆ Try wiggling your ears!

A welcome side-effect of exercising the facial muscles might be to keep wrinkles at bay.

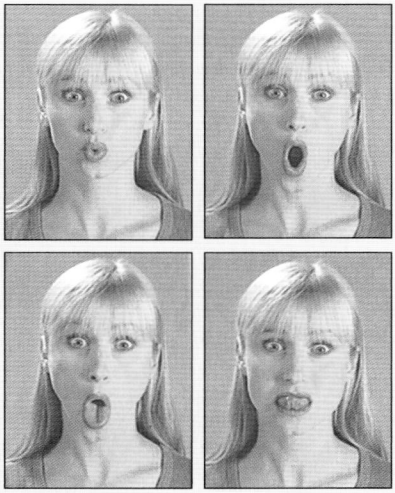

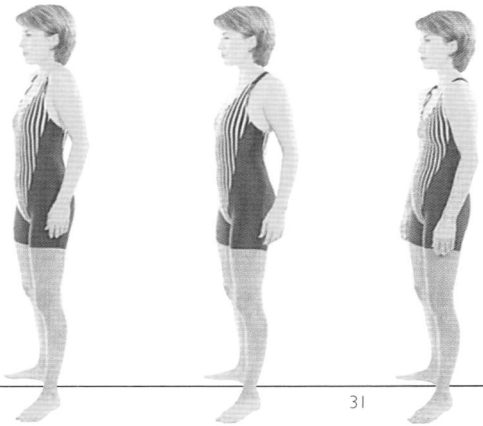

▷ *With arms hanging down, lift your shoulders up, backwards and continuing in a circle.*

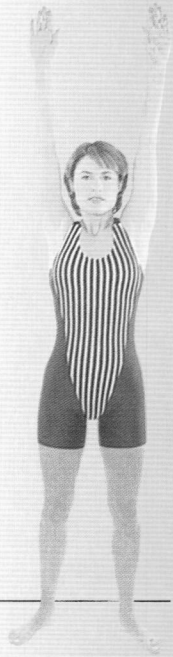

▷ *Stretch your arms as high above your head as you can reach.*

Foot-to-Head Relaxation

The most effective way to relax the whole body starts by deliberately tightening the muscles before releasing them, then focusing on feeling the tension draining away. This can take from five minutes to as long as you like.

You'll need a rug to lie on. Using the same one in the same place each time helps to build up the relaxation habit. Turn up the heating, or put a blanket over you. If you wish, put on a tape of peaceful music without a strong rhythm.

◆ Lie on your back on the floor with feet apart and arms slightly away from the body, palms up. Close your eyes and let your breathing slow down.

◆ Breathe out before you tense each part of your body. Breathe naturally as you lie and feel the relaxation before tensing the next part.

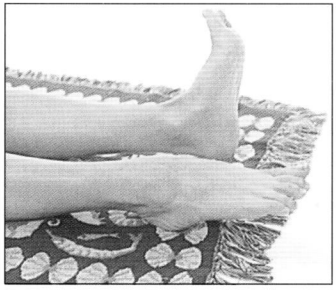

◆ Starting with the left foot, clench your toes, flex the foot with toes upwards and try to tighten every muscle in the foot, lifting it slightly off the floor. Hold this for a few seconds, then relax, letting the foot roll naturally outwards. Feel tension pour out like a liquid soaking through the floor and away. Pause for a moment after relaxing each part of the body to feel this release of tension.

◆ Tighten the calf muscles. Hold this for a few seconds, then relax the calf. Tighten the thigh muscles, feeling tension around the knee as well as the thigh. Hold this for a few seconds, then relax. Feel the relaxation in your whole leg and foot. Now work up the right leg in the same way.

◆ Work your way up the body – buttocks, abdominal muscles, chest and finally upper back, pushing shoulder blades together before releasing them.

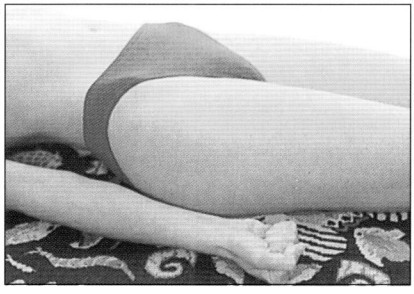

◆ The arms follow the same pattern as the legs. Clench the left fist tightly before releasing, then flex the left arm like a body-builder and relax it, then press the whole arm tightly to the body, tensing the shoulder, and release. Do the same with the right arm, clenching the fists and tensing all the muscles before releasing.

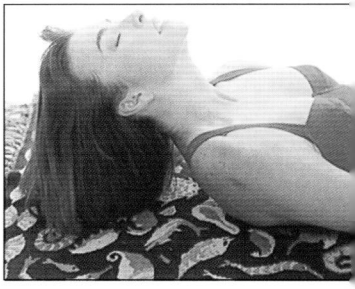

◆ Lift the shoulders and tense the neck as tightly as you can, raising the head slightly, then release.

◆ Clench the teeth, tightly close the eyes and knot up every muscle in the face. Relax with lips slightly parted.

◆ Feel how heavy your head is, sinking into the floor, your whole body perfectly comfortable. Lie peacefully for a few minutes, letting the relaxation spread into every cell of your body.

◆ Then roll onto your side and get up slowly. Stretch your arms high above your head and bring them gently down to your sides as you say to yourself 'I am calm'.

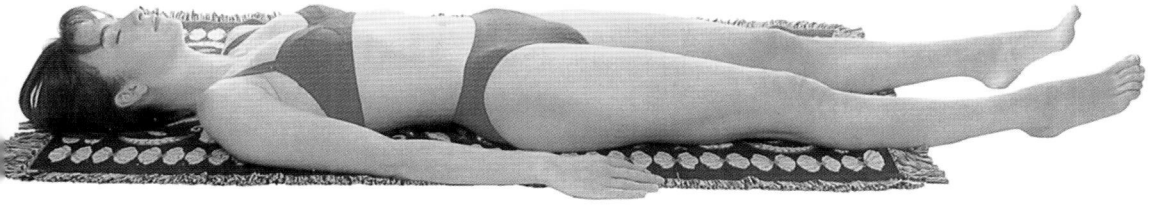

△ *Lie on your back on the floor. Close your eyes and let your breathing slow down. Breathe out and tense each part of your body.*

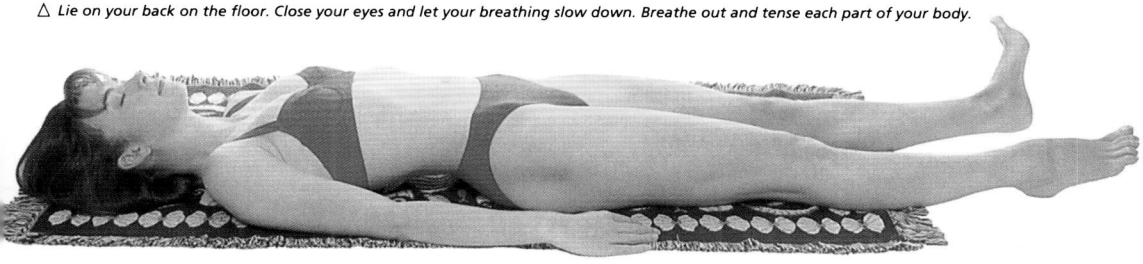

△ *Breathe naturally. Clench and relax your foot, then your calf, working up one leg, then the other.*

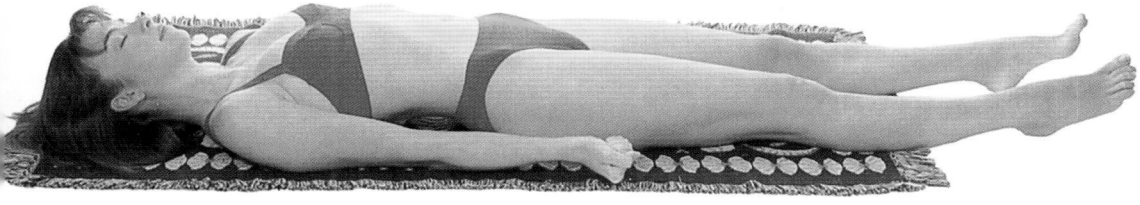

△ *Clench your fist, flex the arm muscles, press tightly to the body and tighten the shoulder. Release then do the same with the other arm.*

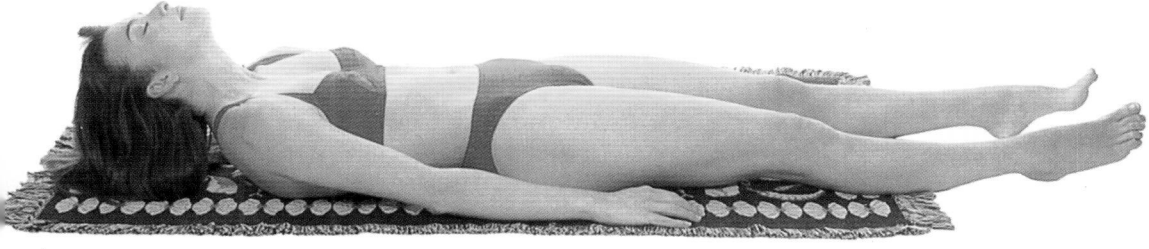

△ *Lift the shoulders and tense your neck as tightly as you can, raising your head slightly, then release.*

SAFE AND SIMPLE

You can also work your way round the body just focusing on each part for a few moments, relaxing it and concentrating on feeling the tension drain away. This is a safer method if you suffer from high blood pressure (make extra-sure you don't hold your breath) or if you have injuries or health problems that make it painful to tense the muscles.

Make Your Own Relaxation Tape

It's often quite hard to concentrate on working your way round your body, especially when you're tired. Lying down, it's easy to doze off. Hearing a voice brings you back to what you're doing. And much as you may need a nap, you'll probably feel better if you stick with the relaxation.

There's a huge variety of relaxation tapes on the market. But you may prefer to hear your own voice with your own choice of background sounds. Bear in mind that if you use recorded background music, say from another tape, legally you may need to pay for permission from the copyright owners, particularly if it could be said to be for public performance.

Decide what length of tape to buy. The foot-to-head relaxation should take at least 10 minutes – remember you're leaving pauses to feel the muscles losing their tension – and you can leave as long as you want at the end to lie and rest.

If you are not using background music throughout, you can end the tape with five minutes relaxing music or nature sounds to bring yourself gently back to wakefulness. On the other side you can record the same text, perhaps with different music, and add the self-hypnosis exercise (see page 70) or instructions for other exercises from this book.

Start with a sound check to make sure you can hear your voice clearly and the music, if any, is at the right level. Make sure you're not going to be interrupted or have distracting background noises.

You will need a stopwatch beside you to time the pauses. As you make your recording, press the 'pause' button rather than stopping if you need to take a break. But don't forget to leave the tape running while you leave the deliberate pauses! Write the name of the exercise and the time it takes to run on the label.

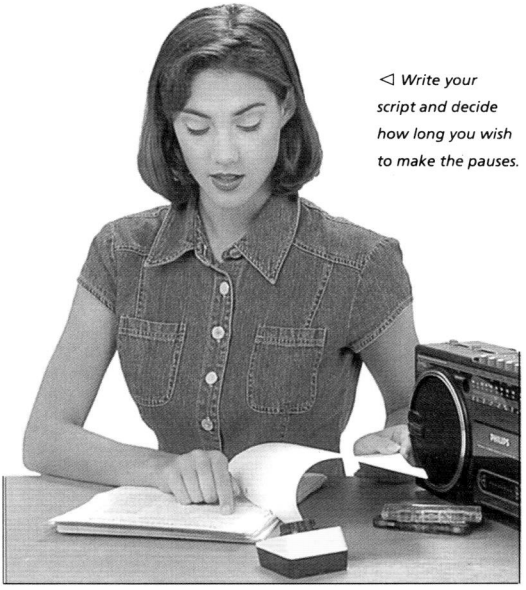

◁ *Write your script and decide how long you wish to make the pauses.*

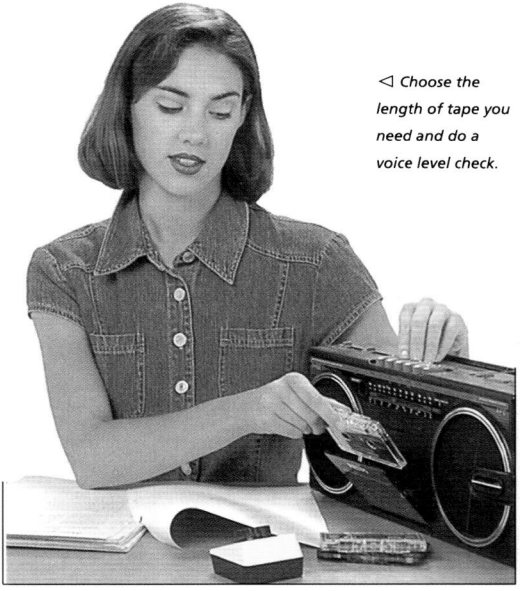

◁ *Choose the length of tape you need and do a voice level check.*

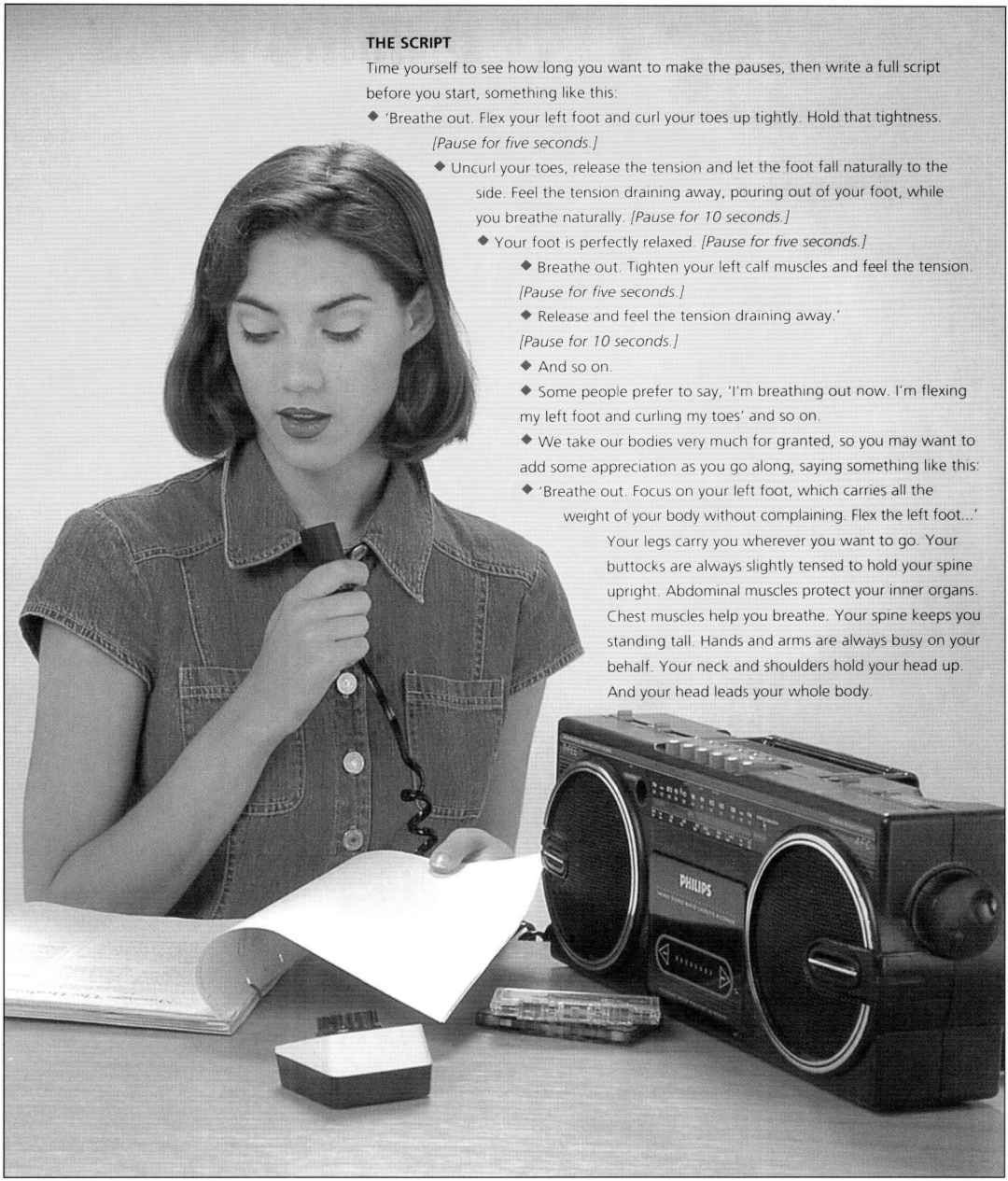

THE SCRIPT

Time yourself to see how long you want to make the pauses, then write a full script before you start, something like this:

- 'Breathe out. Flex your left foot and curl your toes up tightly. Hold that tightness. *[Pause for five seconds.]*
- Uncurl your toes, release the tension and let the foot fall naturally to the side. Feel the tension draining away, pouring out of your foot, while you breathe naturally. *[Pause for 10 seconds.]*
- Your foot is perfectly relaxed. *[Pause for five seconds.]*
- Breathe out. Tighten your left calf muscles and feel the tension. *[Pause for five seconds.]*
- Release and feel the tension draining away.' *[Pause for 10 seconds.]*
- And so on.
- Some people prefer to say, 'I'm breathing out now. I'm flexing my left foot and curling my toes' and so on.
- We take our bodies very much for granted, so you may want to add some appreciation as you go along, saying something like this:
- 'Breathe out. Focus on your left foot, which carries all the weight of your body without complaining. Flex the left foot...' Your legs carry you wherever you want to go. Your buttocks are always slightly tensed to hold your spine upright. Abdominal muscles protect your inner organs. Chest muscles help you breathe. Your spine keeps you standing tall. Hands and arms are always busy on your behalf. Your neck and shoulders hold your head up. And your head leads your whole body.

Massage – The Healing Touch

Massage is one of the oldest forms of healing. It's long been used to break down muscle spasm, improve circulation and help wounds heal. In fact our first instinct, when hurt, is to rub the painful spot.

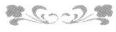

A full body massage by a qualified therapist is a treat. But the basic rubbing and kneading moves are simple enough to learn in a short course or from a book. Get your partner or a friend to learn with you, so you can practice on each other. The moves described here are just a small sample, you can make up more.

All you need are two big towels and some oil or talc. Many shops now sell specially blended massage oil, but in a pinch any vegetable oil will do.

◆ Make sure the room is warm enough for the person being massaged, set the scene and make sure they are comfortable.
◆ Stronger pressure forces knotted muscles to relax, but check it's not hurting.
◆ Use the pads, not the tips, of your fingers and thumbs.
◆ Don't press directly on the spine or joints.
◆ Never massage damaged skin, varicose veins, any inflamed area or a new sprain.
◆ Check with a doctor before massaging anyone with a serious illness (including cancer), hardened arteries or ulcers.

BASIC BACK MASSAGE

Get your partner to undress and lie face down on one of the towels, arms at his sides. Cover him from the waist down with the other towel to keep warm, then put several drops of oil on your palm and rub your hands together.

◆ When your hands are warm, kneel beside your partner with one hand each side of his spine, fingers pointing to his head, and rub your hands in one long movement up to the shoulders, then round and down to cover his back with a fine layer of oil.

◆ Starting from the base of the spine again, rub up beside the spine using your weight to apply more pressure. Hook your hands over his shoulders and pull gently towards you. Bring your hands back down the sides.

◆ The third time up the spine, press into the muscles beside it with the sides of your thumbs, going up a few inches with one and then the other. Go right up the neck, then stroke out across the shoulders.

◆ Find the edges of the shoulder blades and massage along just under them with little thumb circles.

◆ Finish with several long smooth strokes straight up his back, one hand going up as the other returns.

◆ Get him to do the same for you!

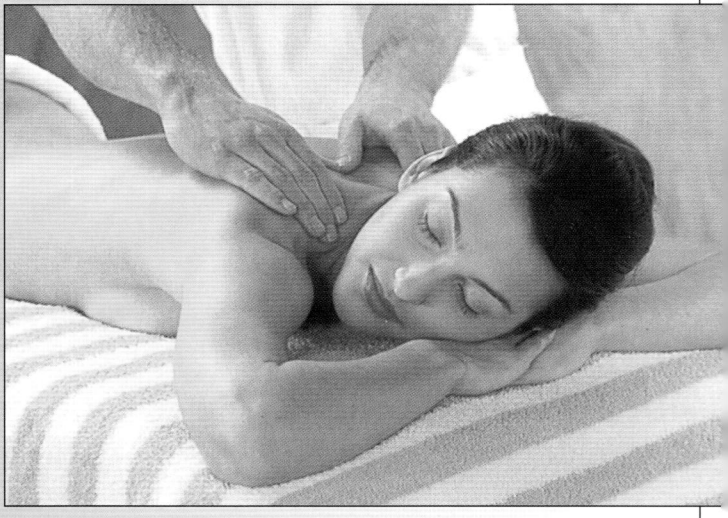

▽ *Spoil yourself with a professional massage occasionally. The soothing movements performed by an expert are not difficult to learn and you will soon be able to practice the techniques at home.*

Simple massage techniques

Any kind of firm rubbing movement will help ease muscle tension and improve circulation.

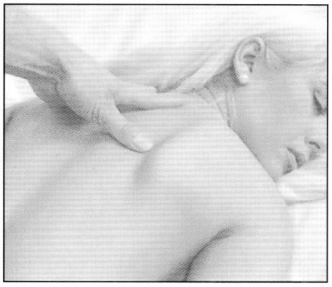

△ *Press the muscles gently, then make small circular movements with the palm of the hand.*

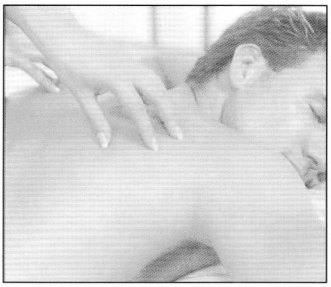

△ *Run your fingers away from you with the lightest of touches of the fingernails.*

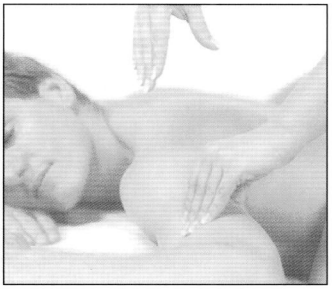

△ *Using both hands in quick succession, pluck lightly over fleshy areas.*

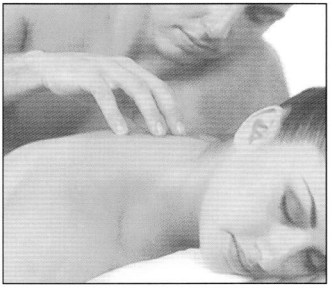

△ *Barely touching, run your fingertips lightly the whole length of the back or limb.*

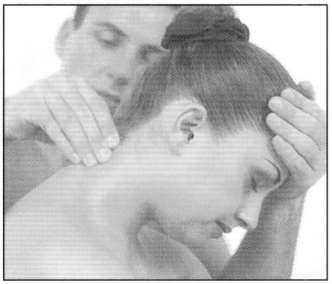

△ *Support the head and gently grip the back of the neck to release tension.*

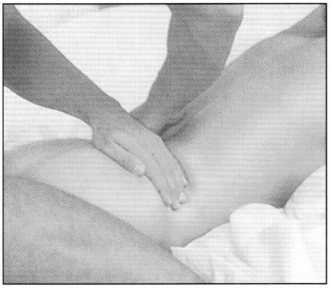

△ *Stroking the muscles will relax and revive. Criss-cross the movements to do both sides.*

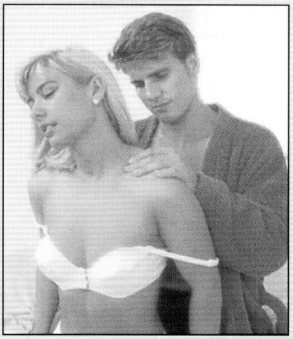

△ *Pick up as much of the flesh as possible and knead it like bread. Press firmly but be careful not to pinch.*

QUICK NECK AND SHOULDER MASSAGE

This is one you can ask your partner to do at the end of a stressful day when you can both relax for the evening. It is just as effective done over clothes – with your friend sitting astride a chair with her back to you. Do each move several times.

◆ Put your forearms on her shoulders and press down.

◆ Pick up the top of the shoulders and knead the muscle, with fingers in front and heels of the hand behind. Continue this movement down the upper arms.

◆ Supporting her head with one hand, put the other on the back of her neck and pull fingers and thumb towards the centre.

◆ Still supporting her head, push up under the edge of her skull with the heel of your hand, working from one side to the other.

◆ While she leans on the back of the chair, massage her back in big circles with the heels of your hands.

Massage Yourself

There's a lot you can do for yourself to unknot aching muscles. Always press with the pads of the fingers, not the tips or nails, and use all four fingers together.

Massage is an excellent way to relieve aches and pains and the stress of everyday life – and even better when you can use the basic techniques to help yourself when you really need them.

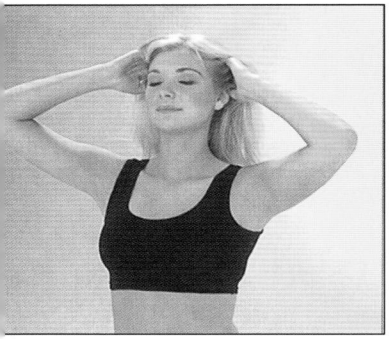

Head

Cup your face in your hands, then slide them back into your hair. Move them in large circles, pressing firmly enough to move the scalp over the skull rather than pulling the hair. Put the heels of your hands on your temples and make the same big circling moves with fingers in the hair.

Then massage all over the scalp with little circling movements (good when you're washing your hair too). Don't forget to rub slowly up behind your ears and gently pull them up, down and back.

All these moves are excellent for easing headaches.

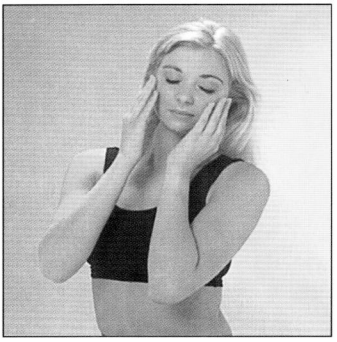

Face

Put all eight fingers on your cheekbones, then, with the pads of your fingers, tap and massage in little circles.

After working on one spot, lift the fingers and move to another without dragging the skin.

Continue down the sides of the face, across the chin and upper lip, then up the cheeks and temples and across the forehead.

Abdomen

Starting just below the navel and heading left, press with your fist in a large circle, anti-clockwise, out towards your side, down to the hip bone, across above the pelvis and back up the side. Repeat the circular movement a few times.

This helps relieve indigestion, but don't press if it hurts.

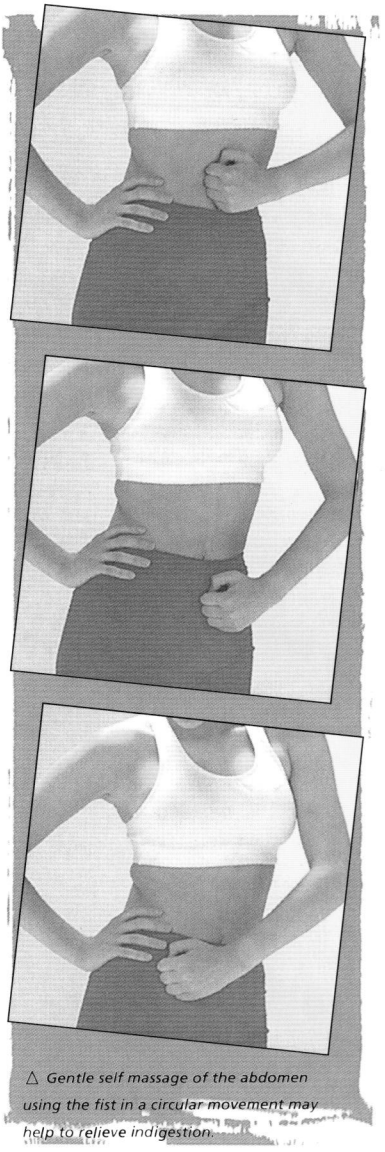

△ *Gentle self massage of the abdomen using the fist in a circular movement may help to relieve indigestion.*

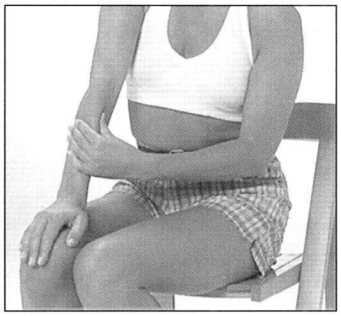

Neck and shoulders

Reach as far down your back as you can, then pull your fingers up beside the spine, pressing hard.

Continue the pressure up to the top of the neck, then massage all over the back of the neck except on the spine.

Massage under the ridge at the base of the skull, from beside the spine to the ears. Line up the fingers one above the other on each side of the spine at the top of the neck.

Press left with the right hand, then right with the left hand, and continue this moving down as far as you can reach. Knead the large shoulder muscles with big pinches.

Hands and arms

With your left hand facing down, put your right hand on top and grip it firmly, kneading the palm, then the fingers. Cup the left hand and knead the palm and joints with the right thumb. Hold and pull each finger in turn, then the thumb. Do the same for the other hand.

Link the fingers and grip the hands together, then try to pull them apart. Squeeze and release all the way up one arm with the other hand. Run your hand up the arm, pressing with the skin between thumb and first finger. Do the same for the other arm.

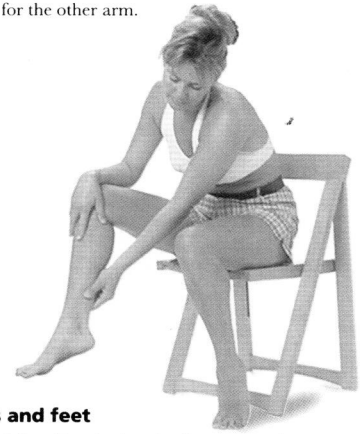

Legs and feet

Knead feet like the hands. Squeeze and rub the calf muscles like the arms, always going up towards the heart. This can help relieve puffy ankles.

Shiatsu – Pressing a Point

Shiatsu, or acupressure, is a kind of acupuncture without needles. It works on the oriental belief that the body's life force circulates like the blood.

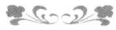

Just as the blood is carried in veins and arteries, the life force – which the Chinese call qi (pronounced 'chee') and the Japanese call ki ('kee') – is believed to circulate in channels called meridians.

Stress, illness, injury or an unhealthy lifestyle can all disrupt the flow. Blocked energy is believed to cause fatigue or jumpiness as well as leading to illness, so shiatsu can be used to help people relax.

Western medical science doesn't recognize this invisible network of meridians, but Chinese and Japanese textbooks include very precise maps. These are what shiatsu practitioners work from when they press particular spots, known as acupressure points, to unblock trapped qi or stimulate the flow.

A weird idea? Well, like Chinese herbal medicine, it's all been written down and practiced for thousands of years. You can try it at home, using steady pressure with the thumb, or a small circular massaging motion over the spot.

To be effective you have to press on exactly the right spot, so if it doesn't work, try visiting a shiatsu therapist. Though it's not always totally painless (that blocked qi can take some pushing along) a trained shiatsu practitioner knows precisely where to press.

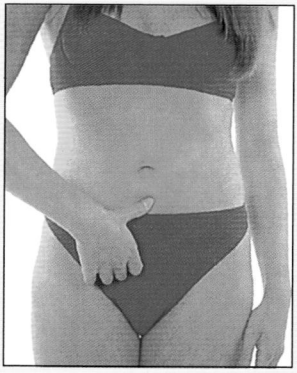

TONING UP

- To strengthen *qi*, press the spot four fingerwidths below the navel.
- For general well-being, press the spot two to three fingerwidths towards the thumb from the outer end of the crease made when the elbow is bent at right angles. This also eases tired arms and legs.

▷ *Press the point between the eyebrows to relieve stress and headaches.*

HELPFUL POINTS

Press or massage the following points for at least 10 seconds.

◆ Anxiety. The little dip below the outer side of the knee, three fingerwidths down from the kneecaps.

◆ Exhaustion. Pinch the front top joint of your little finger, right on the joint itself. Also, press the centre of the palm or the central crease in the ball of the foot.

◆ Insomnia. Squeeze the ear lobes between finger and thumbs.

◆ Craving for a cigarette. Press hard on the 'salt cellar' bone between the collarbones for as long as you can – press down onto the bone, not into your throat.

◆ Racing thoughts and headaches. Massage the natural dip at the temples, about an inch back from the outer edge of your eyes.

◆ Stress and headaches. The point between the eyebrows.

◆ Headaches. Under the ridge at the back of your skull, press into both sides at the same time.

◆ Eye strain. The edge of the nose beside the tear ducts.

◆ Backache. The middle of the crease behind the knee.

◆ Menopausal symptoms. The tip of the chin, right in the centre.

◆ Menstrual problems. A point in the middle of your forehead, three fingerwidths above the eyebrows.

◆ Sharp pain. Rhythmically press the centre of the upper lip. And be sure to see your doctor!

◆ Long-term pain. A point on the back of your hand, three fingerwidths down from the space between ring and little fingers.

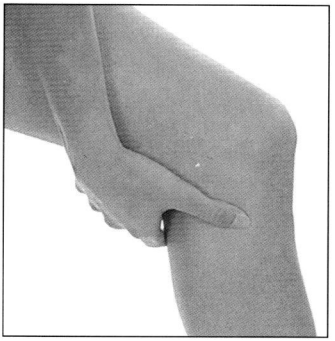

△ *Anxiety – the right spot near the knee.*

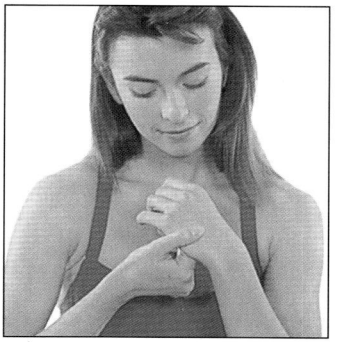

△ *Long-term pain – the back of the hand.*

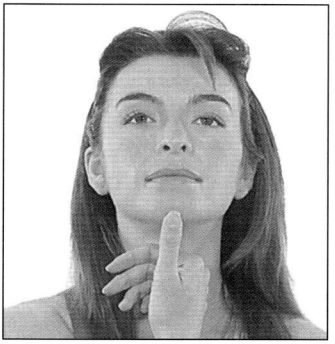

△ *Menstrual problems – the tip of the chin.*

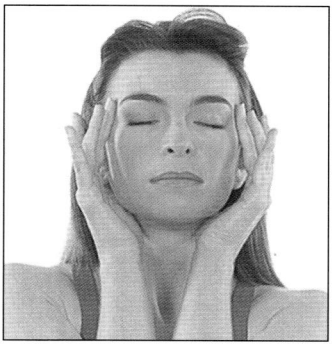

△ *Headaches – massage the temples.*

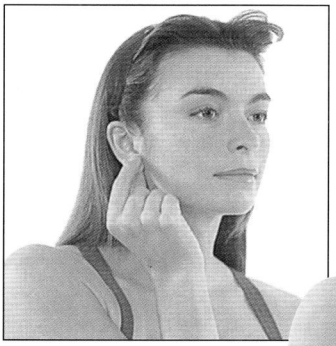

△ *Insomnia.*

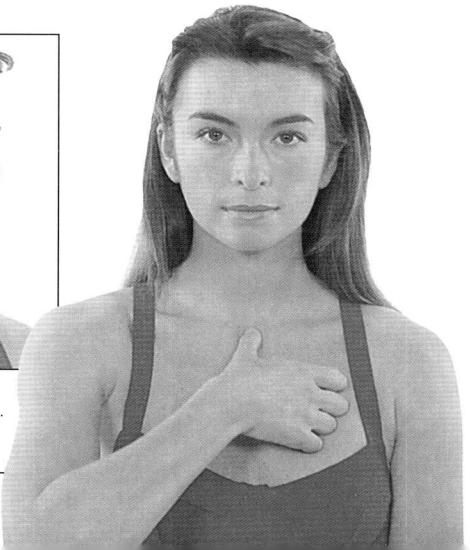

▷ *Cigarette craving .*

Aromatherapy – Healing Scents

We don't use our sense of smell much in the modern world – maybe that's why it can have such a strong effect. Yet aromatic oils have been used in healing for thousands of years. More recently our grandmothers inhaled eucalyptus to cure colds and massaged their temples with lavender to ease headaches. These days aromatherapists generally use essential oils as part of a healing massage.

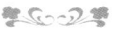

Scientists have now started discovering how different scents affect the brain. Medical tests measuring brain activity have found lavender helps people relax, for example, while jasmine makes them more alert.

Try before you buy and choose the scents you like best – your brain responds more strongly to these. You can use them alone or make up your own recipes. Don't worry if one you find soothing is described somewhere else as 'stimulating' – some,

ESSENTIAL SAFETY

Essential oils can have powerful effects. If you're pregnant, don't use (from these lists) cedarwood, clary sage, cypress, jasmine, juniper, myrrh, marjoram or valerian. Avoid camomile, geranium, lavender and rose in the first three months of pregnancy.

- If you suffer from conditions such as epilepsy or high blood pressure, consult an aromatherapist through one of the organizations listed on pages 94 and 95 before using essential oils.
- If an oil irritates your skin – though those on these lists should all be safe – wash it off at once.

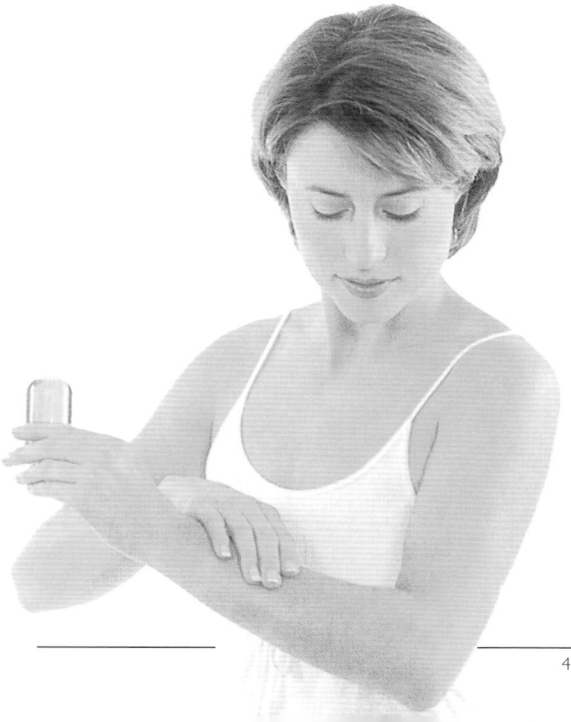

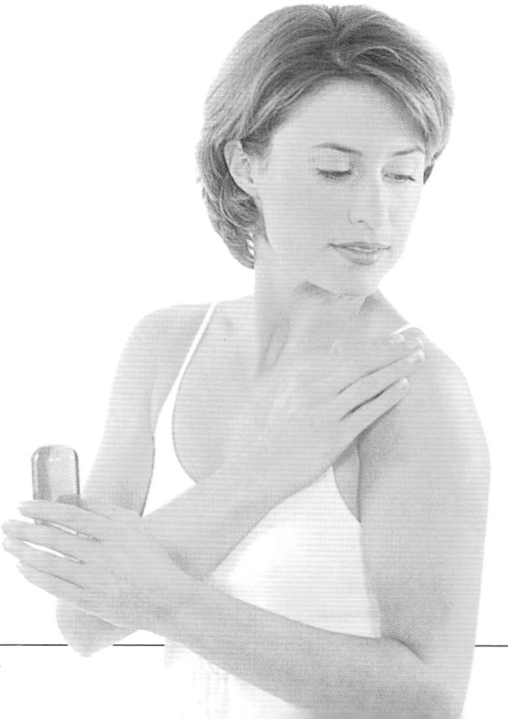

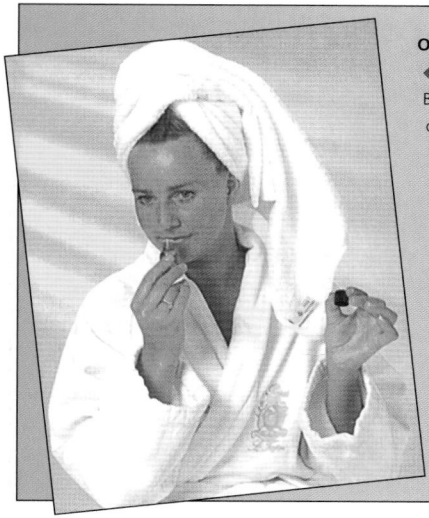

OILS TO EASE YOUR MIND

◆ *Relaxing*

Bay, benzoin, bois de rose, cajeput, calamus, calendula, camomile, caraway, carrot seed, clary sage, cypress, frankincense, geranium, hawthorn, heliotrope, jasmine, juniper, lavender, lime, marigold, marjoram, melissa, neroli, opoponax, patchouli, petitgrain, rose, rosewood, sandalwood, taget, valerian, vanilla, vetivert, violet leaf, yarrow, ylang ylang.

◆ *Remedies for shock*

Camomile, cedarwood, geranium, lavender, melissa, neroli, rose.

◆ *To aid sleep*

Benzoin, camomile, clary sage, cypress, frankincense, geranium, jasmine, juniper, lavender, melissa, myrrh, myrtle, neroli, patchouli, rose, sandalwood, ylang ylang.

◁ *Take time to try a few different essential oils before you buy the ones you prefer.*

like rose and neroli, may stimulate the brain but soothe the nerves at the same time. Others balance the emotions, calming or stimulating as needed – these include geranium, rosewood and valerian.

◆ Treat yourself to a massage by an aromatherapist, or swap with a friend, using techniques from the massage section. Add two or three drops of essential oil to each teaspoonful of vegetable oil such as grapeseed, sunflower, safflower or soya.

◆ Electric or candle-fuelled oil burners spread the scent through a room. This is also a subtle way of treating children.

◆ Add half a dozen drops of essential oil to bath water as you get in. It remains effective for up to 20 minutes.

◁ *You will instinctively choose the oils which you find most appealing. These are likely to to do you the most good.*

▷ *Your favourite and most effective fragrances can be incorporated into your everyday beauty routine.*

How do you know it's a real essential oil?

Ready mixed bath or burning oils are handy for everyday use. But to get the strongest effects you need unblended essential oils. These tend to be thin, strong-smelling, quick to evaporate – and more expensive than cheaper 'essential oils' which are probably already blended. Keep oils in dark glass containers, away from heat and sunlight, with caps screwed on tightly.

Reflexology – Body and Sole

The idea behind reflexology is that the whole body is represented in the foot, so pressing a certain part of the sole has an effect on the corresponding part of the body. Some people claim the same is true of the hands and even of the ear lobes.

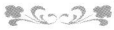

Reflexologists say they find a crunchy feeling like grains under their fingers while massaging the foot, if there's something wrong with the part of the body that spot represents – so they press harder to break it down. This way, they can safely tackle spinal injuries or internal organs, though a professional reflexology session may be quite uncomfortable in places.

It's been proved effective in treating premenstrual syndrome, and not only because any kind of massage makes people feel better – it was tested against an ordinary foot massage. Some hospitals now offer it to patients after surgery.

Reflexology – Hitting the spot

Anyone can do a wonderfully relaxing foot massage, rubbing and kneading with a little cream or oil and pulling the toes. Just press firmly enough not to tickle! A professional will do the best job – but here are some points to try.

- Hold the foot firmly, and press your thumbs into any point that needs massaging. You can also massage in small circular movements.
- Use the rounded pads of your fingers or thumbs above the top joint (short nails are best). Don't massage over broken skin or injuries.

Relax and revive

Run your finger along the ball of your foot, furthest from the toes, and you'll find a natural curve as if two sections were joined. Find the spot in that curve just below the ball of the foot and nearly halfway across from the inner edge, and keep pressing with your thumb to massage the solar plexus point.

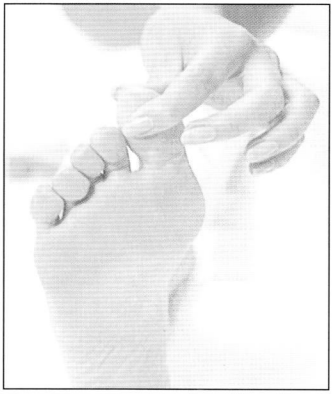

Headaches

Squeeze all over the pad of the big toe – this is also said to stimulate the brain (*see above*). If a headache is caused by sinuses, squeeze the sides and back of each toe. A tired headache across the forehead can be eased by pressing just below the big toenail.

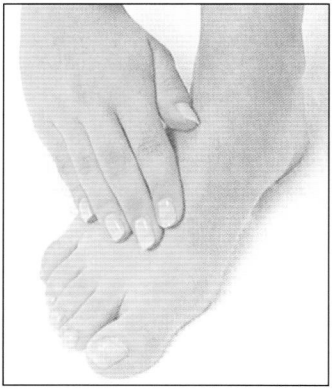

PMS

The womb point is halfway between the bottom of the inside ankle bone and the point of the heel. The ovaries are in the same spot on the outside of the foot and the fallopian tubes are represented by a line running across the top of the foot joining the ankle bones. You could also press the pituitary gland spot, at the bottom of the big toe pad, right in the middle (*see below*).

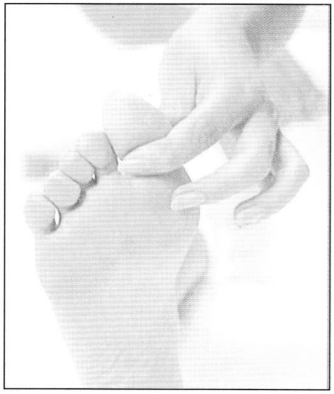

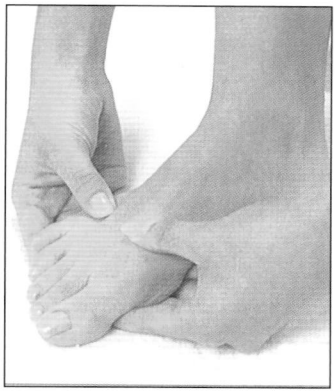

Sore breasts

Gently rub up and down the top of the foot, covering a couple of inches from the base of the toes (*see left*).

Aching shoulders

Holding the foot in both hands, knead and massage your way across both top and sole about an inch from the toes.

Backache

The big toe represents your head, so the spine runs all the way down the inside edge of the foot. Pressing and kneading all the way down could ease tired back muscles.

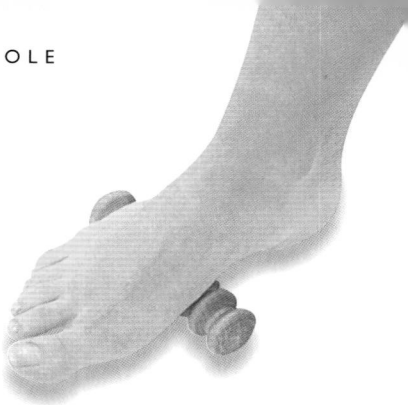

△ *Wooden foot massagers are now widely available and can be very effective.*

▽ *An experienced reflexologist may be able to diagnose and treat problem areas.*

The Alexander Technique

Remember, as a child, being prodded in the back and told to stand up straight? Yet standing up straight, to most adults, means lifting the chin, throwing the shoulders back and the spine forward at the waist – a rigid, unnatural posture. The rest of the time, we slouch. Either way, we're putting a cruel strain on the spine – which has enough to contend with trying to keep us upright.

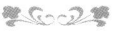

The Alexander Technique is named after a young Australian actor who, at the turn of the century, found his voice becoming weak and hoarse. Doctors couldn't help, and resting only worked till he went back on stage. Finally he realized his tense, stiff-backed posture was crushing his vocal cords – and damaging his whole body. Starting by curing his own problem, he worked out a series of exercises to break the bad habits of a lifetime.

It sounds like hard work, but it's actually about making movement easier. For most of us, the way we stand and move now is a lot more effort than it should be. Our backs ache, our shoulders knot up with tension.

Getting up from a seat, we tip our heads back or push off with our hands instead of letting the powerful leg muscles lift us forward in one easy, fluid movement. We stand with the pelvis tipped forward, one leg taking the weight, one shoulder leading – it seems natural simply because we've grown used to it, but it takes far more effort than is necessary. But once you've learned the easy way to do things, you may wonder how you could have made all that effort every day.

There are books on the subject, but it's really worth taking one-to-one tuition or, more economically, group classes. A teacher can correct oddities that you were not aware of.

Let the tension run out

- Lie on your back on a carpeted floor, with a pile of paperback books beside you.
- Put the books under your head, experimenting till your neck is straight rather than tipped back (as it would be without any support) or forward. This usually takes more books than you'd think – a pile anything up to four or five inches high, depending on how rounded your shoulders are. As your posture improves, you won't need so many.
- Raise your knees slightly so the small of the back sinks naturally to the floor. Gently bring one knee at a time up to your chest for 10 seconds, then shuffle your bottom further along the floor to lengthen the spine. With feet on the floor, shoulder-width apart, keep the knees comfortably raised.
- You may find it easiest to rest your toes against a wall to stop them sliding. Rest your hands on your lower abdomen and relax for at least 10 minutes. Get up by rolling onto your side, then your knees.
- Sometimes this may make the lower back ache temporarily, but don't give up – it's the muscles starting to let go of long-held tension.

◁ *It may take more paperback books than you think, but as your posture improves you will not need so many.*

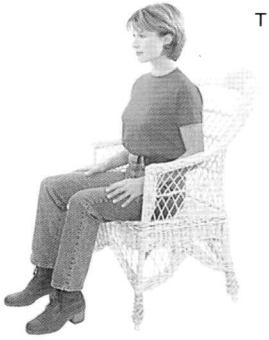

△ *Hands off the chair arms – so you are not hunching your shoulders.*

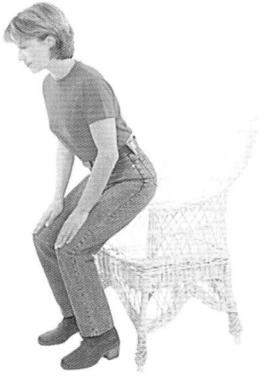

△ *Allow your powerful leg muscles to take the strain. It's what they're for!*

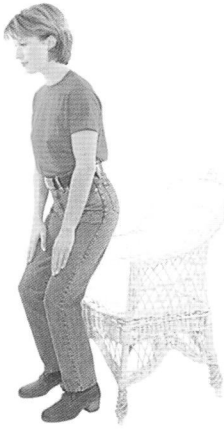

△ *Keep your spine straight with head and neck aligned at all times. Do not throw your head up or backwards.*

△ *Look in a mirror – it's surprising how off-centre most of us are. Learning better posture takes a huge strain off our bodies.*

Yoga – Your Flexible Friend

It's not just about strange postures and enviably supple spines. Yoga is now credited with relieving a host of diseases and it's probably the most popular form of exercise for relaxation.

Yoga does more than just improve flexibility, important though that is – it is believed to have an effect on the hormones and, by emphasizing correct breathing, improves the oxygen supply to the whole body. Most classes include breathing exercises and relaxation as well as the asanas or poses.

Like meditation, yoga is sometimes mistaken for some kind of cult. Wrong in both cases – religions may use these techniques, just as Christian church-goers sing and eat bread – but they're also just healthy things to do.

Easy yoga postures

The help of a good teacher is important, as it's often difficult to tell if your position is slightly out of line. But these simple asanas can help with tiredness, backache and stress.

The Pose of a Child

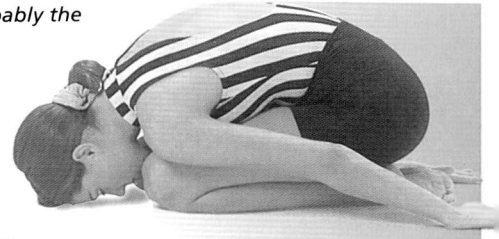

The Pose of a Child
Very restful, especially for a tired back. Kneeling on your heels, lean forward as far as you can and place your forehead on the floor. Rest your face on a cushion if you can't reach the floor. Let your arms lie beside your legs, palms up. Stay as long as you like, breathing normally.

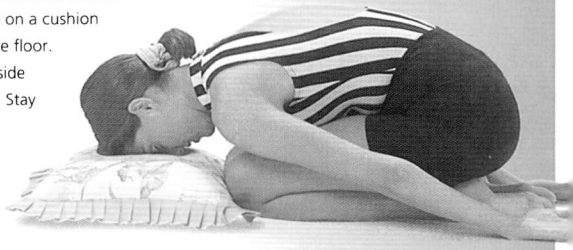

The Inverted Corpse
Never mind the name – it's wonderful when you're tired. If anyone asks, it's your yoga homework. Just lie on your back near a wall and rest your feet a short distance up the wall, legs together. It's good for varicose veins too, but don't do it if you have high blood pressure.

The Inverted Corpse

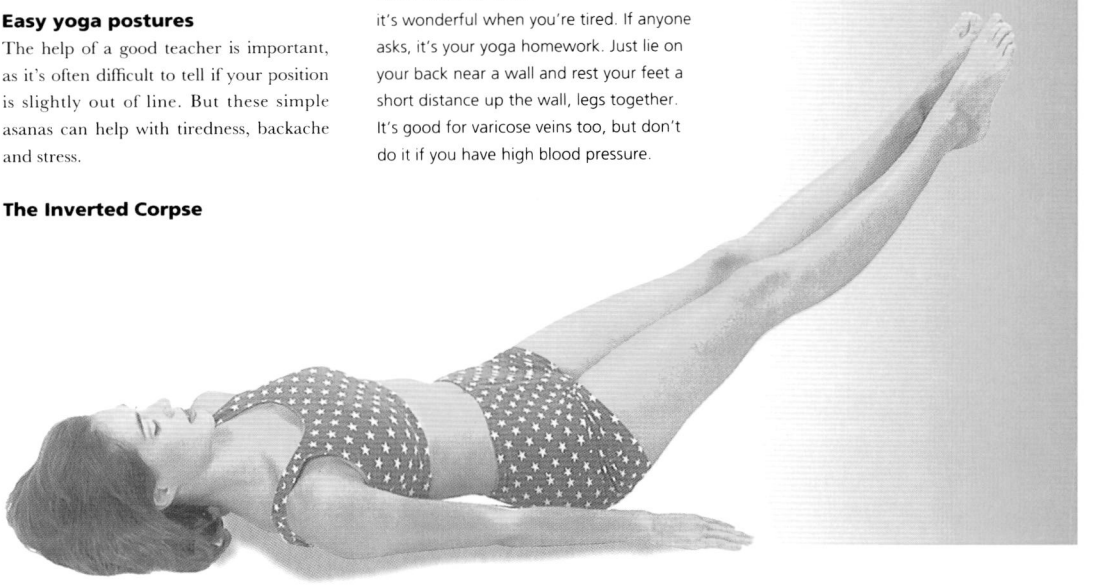

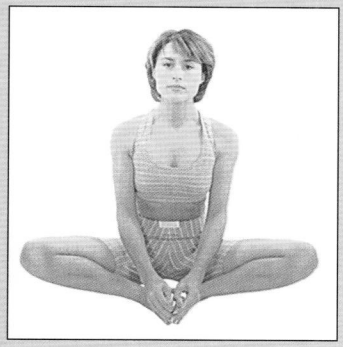

△ *Performed as a warm up exercise for the Lotus position, the Butterfly begins with spine erect and soles of the feet together, close to the body.*

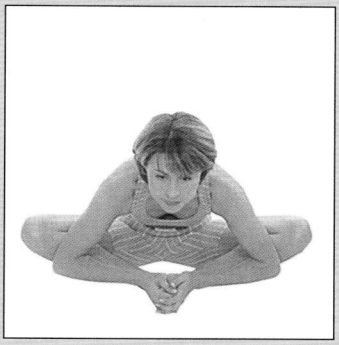

△ *Carefully lean forward, clasping the feet with both hands. Keep movements slow and breathing steady. Lotus warm-up exercises increase hip, knee and ankle flexibility.*

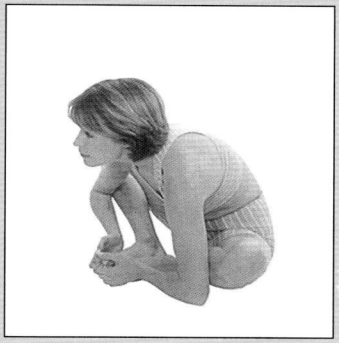

△ *Lean forward gently, do not over stretch to begin with. Sit up, clasp the feet, move the knees up and down like the wings of a butterfly then press the knees to the floor.*

SAFETY FIRST

- Yoga can reduce high blood pressure but certain postures could be dangerous – see your doctor first.
- It's best on an empty stomach.
- Avoid head and neck stands if you have back trouble.
- Don't stay in a position if it hurts.
- Tell your teacher if you have a medical condition.
- Avoid anything that feels dangerous.

The Mountain

Sitting, preferably with legs crossed in front of you, inhale and raise your arms above your head, close to your ears, palms together. Stretch upwards for as long as it feels comfortable, breathing naturally. Breathe out as you bring them down.

The Harmless Cobra

The cobra usually involves coming up onto your hands and arching your spine with your head tipped back. The harmless cobra is a more spine-friendly version. Lying on your front with your face on the floor, put your elbows on the floor beside you at shoulder-level, fingers pointing forwards. Lift your head and come smoothly up onto your elbows, facing ahead. Push your ribs forward to feel the stretch in your spine.

Smart moves

Yoga can be strenuous, especially if you're stiff or unfit, and some postures put a lot of pressure on joints or the spine.

If you have back problems or find ordinary yoga too demanding, look for specialist classes, which often have names like 'yoga therapy'. Some organizations train instructors in the use of yoga to treat physical problems – not only back pain but diseases like asthma and multiple sclerosis.

The Harmless Cobra

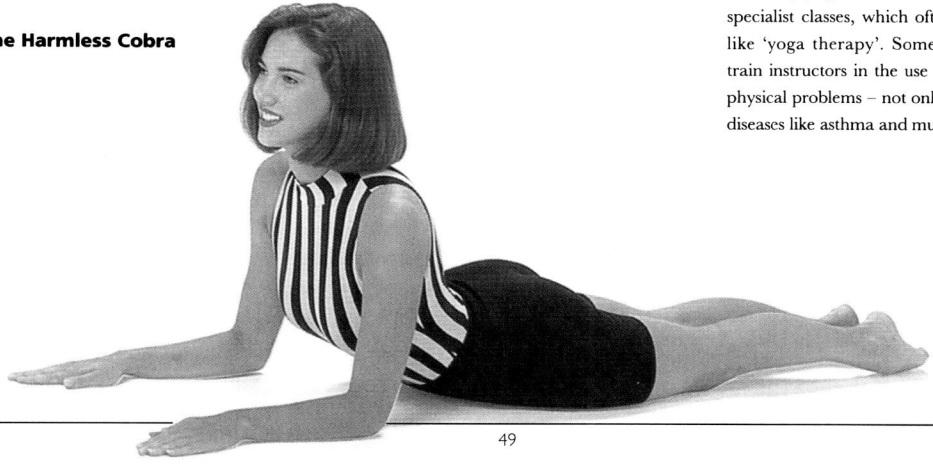

T'ai Chi – Chinese Serenity

Have you ever seen pictures of hundreds of people practising slow, ballet-like exercises together in a Chinese park as the sun comes up through the mist? You can still see this any morning in towns and cities across that vast country. They're doing t'ai chi (or tai ji quan), probably the most peaceful, graceful form of exercise ever invented.

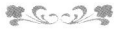

Surprisingly, t'ai chi started out as a martial art! Developed more than 400 years ago, this calming technique now forms part of Chinese astronauts' training. According to traditional theory, t'ai chi tackles illness by balancing the *qi* – the body's energy or life force.

To a westerner, the most obvious benefits are in lowering blood pressure, relieving chest disease, improving flexibility and bringing a profound sense of tranquillity.

T'ai chi is so pleasing that you don't need huge motivation to practise – it's very satisfying when you can glide through the whole sequence, or even a section. The only thing you need is a bit of space. The sequence covers several yards, which is one reason why people practise outdoors.

If you haven't quite got the nerve to glide across the local park, don't be put off. Just use the longest space you can find, adding a neat turn whenever you reach a wall. If your home's the right shape, you could leave doors open and work your way out of the living room, down the hall and into the kitchen.

Less strenuous than yoga, t'ai chi can be done by practically anyone. Even in a wheelchair you could do the upper body movements. As weight-bearing exercise, it helps keep the brittle-bone disease osteoporosis at bay after the menopause.

There are several styles, taking from five to 25 minutes, and some are practised with bent legs. If this is hard on your knees try one of the others or simply continue without bending so deeply – it's not vital.

Balancing the qi

- It's best to learn t'ai chi in a class or from a video, though there are some useful books as back-up.
- In these preparatory exercises, you start by standing with knees comfortably loose and back straight.
- Always breathe fully, into your abdomen, in time with the movements.

▽ *T'ai chi is a form of spiritual meditation, working on the principles of the constant flow of movement. Stand in a relaxed stance, transferring weight from one foot to the other whilst breathing in rhythm.*

Flowing Moves

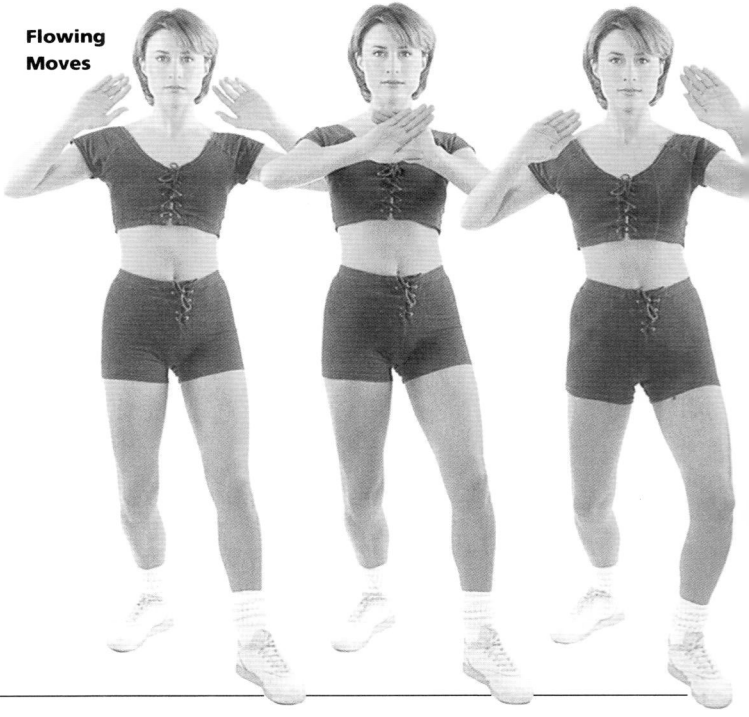

T'ai chi rod

◆ Focus on your 'centre', the point just below your navel.

◆ Hold a 12-inch ruler between your palms in front of your abdomen, parallel to the ground.

◆ Slowly move it a few inches up, out, down and back towards you, making smooth circles.

◆ You can also do this while walking, one circle for each step.

Qi gong march, bouncing ball

◆ As you breathe in, bend the right elbow and slowly lift the hand, keeping the wrist loose and palm down, to shoulder-level.

◆ Raise the opposite knee at the same time. Look straight ahead.

◆ As you breathe out, bring down the hand as if bouncing a ball in slow motion, and bring down the foot at the same time.

◆ Breathe in, raising the other hand and foot.

◆ Repeat 10 times or more, when you are tired.

Exercise – Dump Your Stress

It's something most of us feel guilty about not doing enough. Yet working up a sweat is a guaranteed route to relaxation. Aerobic exercise – that's anything that speeds up your heartbeat, not necessarily an aerobics class – increases the brain's output of endorphins, which give a natural high.

Lively exercise improves whatever mood you're in – if you're depressed it'll cheer you up, and if you're fine it'll leave you feeling dynamic. It also works off harmful stress hormones. And the fitter you get through regular exercise, the better your body can cope with stress.

Gentle methods based on increasing flexibility help in a different way, calming and lowering blood pressure. If you're out of shape, start slowly with a daily walk. You can always wear an unrevealing tracksuit if you progress to fitness classes – anyway, everyone else is too concerned about their own shape to notice yours!

See what's on at local sports and leisure centres, gyms, colleges and evening classes, then choose something you enjoy at a level that's not too hard (if you're constantly struggling, you're more likely to injure yourself or give up). If you fancy aerobics but don't enjoy one class, try someone else's. Look out for unusual activities, like circus skills or ethnic dance classes that sound like fun.

What's your style?

Think what you'd enjoy most, and what you don't want. Swimming's out, for example, if you need something you can do in odd spare minutes. If you're not likely to be free at the same time every week, avoid new skills you have to learn in a class. If you need to be highly controlled and organized in your everyday life, give yoga a miss and go dancing.

▽ *If you are new to exercise classes, choose an activity where you can work out at your own pace, or start off at home with a video.*

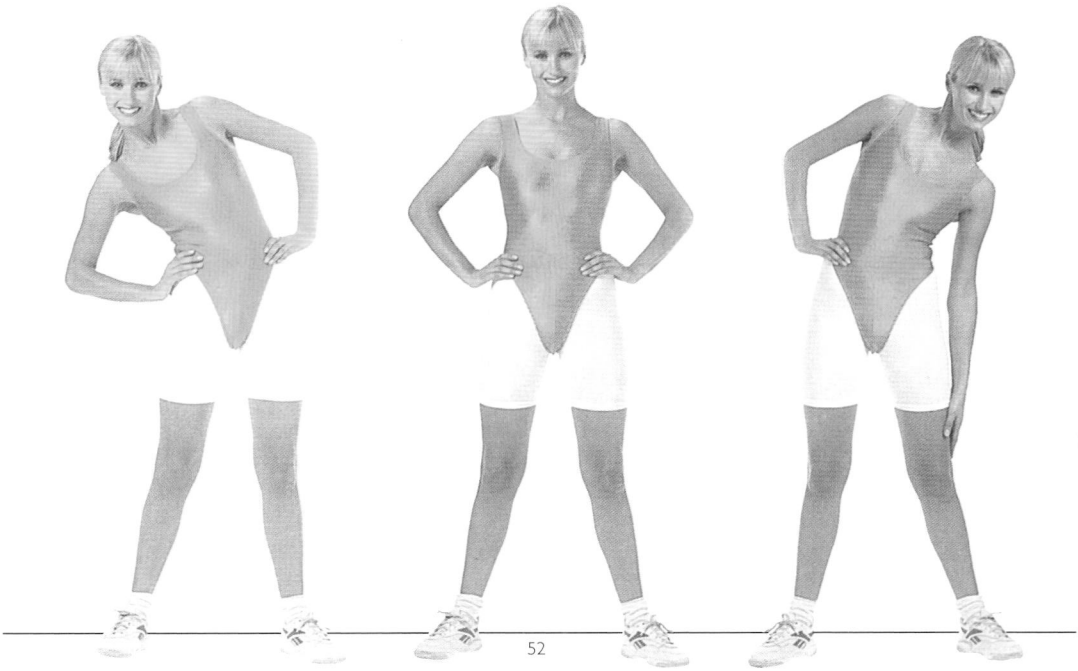

DO YOU WANT:

Activities with music? Dancing, aerobics and the wealth of other fitness classes now available such as sliding, stepping and spinning (group exercise-biking).

To make friends? Rowing, team sports, and there's a possibility with any classes, of course. With team games, you'll need to make a regular commitment to your fellow team mates.

Something you can do alone? Running, power-walking, skipping, exercise-biking, skating, cycling, swimming, exercise videos. If you get bored, or feel a lack of encouragement, join a club or work out with a friend.

A new skill? Martial arts, dance, fencing, gymnastics, acrobatics. You'll need perseverance – and be willing to take a few falls.

Outdoor activities? Canoeing, climbing, rambling, orienteering, skiing. You can get cold, wet and possibly hurt, but not bored.

Something not too strenuous? Circle dancing, swimming, T'ai chi, Yoga and similar gentle movement classes.

Something demanding? Boxing workouts, martial arts, some team games, outdoor activities (some leisure centres also have indoor climbing walls), advanced fitness classes.

Partner activities? Tennis, table tennis, badminton, squash – get a friend to join you. Best if you're at similar levels.

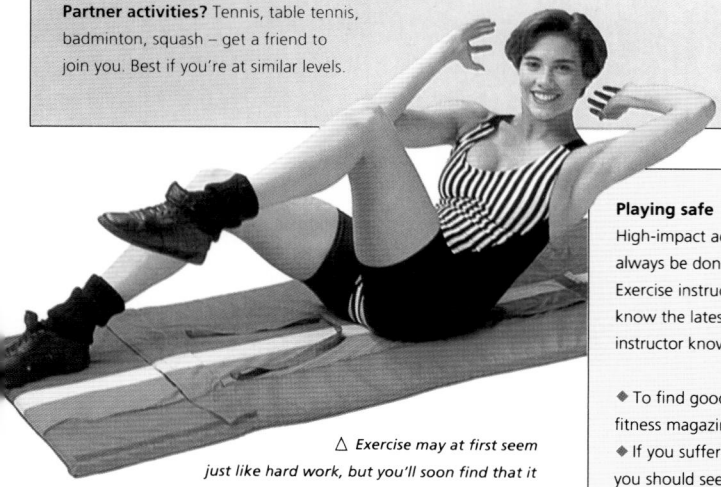

△ *Exercise may at first seem just like hard work, but you'll soon find that it can be good fun at the same time as being good for you!*

Playing safe

High-impact aerobics (with running or jumping moves) should always be done in a gym with a purpose built sprung floor. Exercise instructors should have formal qualifications and they'll know the latest about safe and effective exercises. Let the instructor know if you have any health problems.

◆ To find good, safe videos, read the reviews in health and fitness magazines.

◆ If you suffer from any illness, especially high blood pressure, you should see your doctor before taking up exercise.

Stretch – Relaxing Like a Cat

One of the first ways stress shows itself in our bodies is through stiff, knotted muscles that eventually stop us moving freely. Stretching is a simple way to release the tension. It's a good way to start the morning or to follow a foot-to-head relaxation and is valuable before and after exercise. Just watch a cat or dog enjoying a long, all-body stretch – tension never gets a look-in.

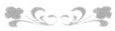

When you're stretching, never make fast or jerky movements, bounce, or try to force a stretch too far. You can stretch more by breathing out as you make the effort, breathing in and then gently leaning a little further into it as you breathe out again.

All these stretches are done standing up – straight but not stiff or arching the back – unless otherwise specified. Hold each one for five to 10 seconds and repeat a few times. When you've stretched one side or limb, do the other too. You can also include some of the upper-body relaxers on page 30.

◆ Do some big waking-up stretches – arms up over head and out to the side as far back as they'll go, stretching out to the tips of your fingers. You can do this lying down too, stretching your legs out and down as far as they will go.

◆ Tilt your head sideways till your ear is near your left shoulder (*see above*), then do the same the other side, then let your chin sink onto your chest.

◆ Stretch arms out in front, interlacing

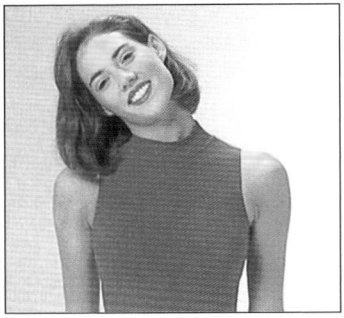

△ *Tilt your head sideways.*

◁ *Do some big waking-up stretches.*

▽ *Stretch your arms out in front, interlacing your fingers. Raise your arms above your head and back as far as they will comfortably go.*

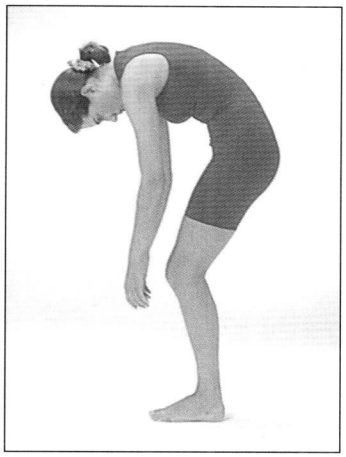

△ *Uncurl vertebra by vertebra.*

◆ Standing on one leg, pull the other foot up to your buttocks, being extra-careful not to arch your back (*see right*).

◆ Take a short step forward then bend your knees as if curtsying, but keeping heels on the ground.

◆ Standing straight with feet shoulder-width apart, relax the spine by bending forward and letting the head hang down, with legs slightly bent, arms dangling. Straighten up slowly, vertebra by vertebra, unrolling from the bottom of your spine very gradually up to the top (*see left*). If you lose your balance you can try this leaning against a wall, or with the help of a friend, but if you experience dizziness leave this exercise out.

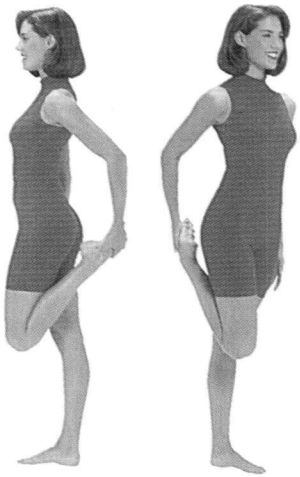

△ *Pull the foot up to your buttocks.*

fingers and turning palms outwards. Raise above head and back as far as they comfortably go (*see opposite page*).

◆ Roll both shoulders backwards in big circles (*see pictures page 31*).

◆ Keeping your spine straight and hips still, put both hands on your left hip and turn your whole body from the waist to look over your left shoulder, pushing gently with your hands (see right).

◆ On hands and knees, hump your back as high as you can, head down, then stretch with back straight, head level, so the spine continues in a straight line up to the skull. (Don't do this if you suffer from epilepsy.)

◆ Sit on the floor with legs splayed out, knees soft – don't try to push the legs down flat or lock the knees. Lean towards your right ankle, trying to keep your spine straight and leaning up out of the hips.

◆ Rotate and flex your feet and wiggle the toes.

▷ *Keep your spine straight and turn your whole body from the waist.*

Walk Away From Your Troubles

Walking combines proven stress relief with the easiest, most convenient form of exercise and the cheapest way of getting around. Try to take a walk every day, even just for 10 minutes – in your lunch break, instead of short car journeys or by getting off the bus a couple of stops earlier. Most relaxing of all is a long country walk with a picnic – and water – in your backpack.

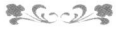

It's best to wear lace-up walking shoes or trainers and start with some leg stretches. But don't worry if circumstances aren't perfect, any walk will do you good.

◆ Set out at a stroll for the first five to 10 minutes. Walk tall, with shoulders relaxed and your back straight but not stiff. Breathe deeply. If you like, try to relax each part of your body on the way, as in the Safe and Simple foot-to-head relaxation – 'My left foot feels perfectly relaxed' and so on.

◆ Start noticing your surroundings. Enjoy front gardens of houses. Feel the bark of trees. Really look at the texture and colour of old brick walls. Smell flowers. Listen to all the surrounding noises and start distinguishing sounds – birdsong, traffic, voices, footsteps, radios, animals.

◆ Speed up till you're walking briskly, breathing harder and swinging your arms. At this speed, it's good aerobic exercise.

▽ ***Any walk is beneficial to your health – in breathtaking countryside or to the local shop.***

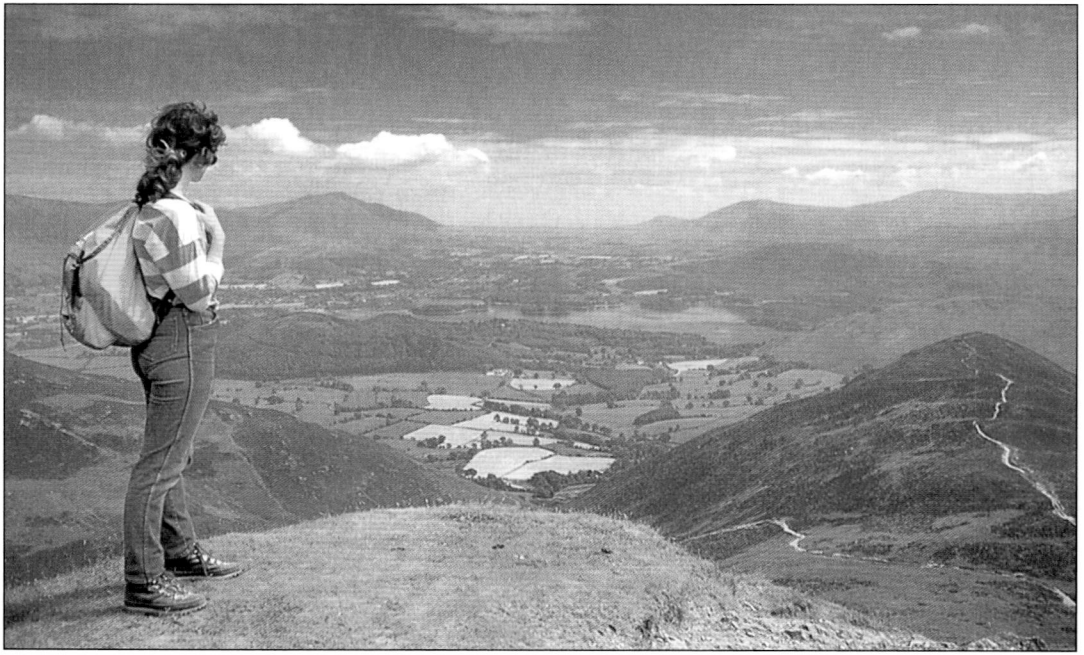

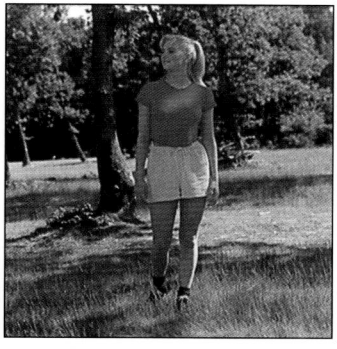

△ *Start noticing your surroundings...feel the bark of trees...smell flowers...listen to all the surrounding noises.*

◆ As you get fitter, you could combine walking with patches of jogging or pump your arms like a race-walker. You shouldn't be gasping – keep to a pace at which you could just about hold a conversation.
◆ Slow down to a comfortable stroll for the last five or 10 minutes, to avoid cramps and slowly bring breathing and heart rate back to normal.

Walking back to happiness

◆ Any time you feel like screaming, get out and walk fast for a few minutes till you've cooled down a bit. Help this along by breathing as deeply and slowly as you can. Put your upset out of your mind as soon as possible – concentrate on your movement and breathing. Then slow down and do the rest of the walking exercise.

Mind and body

◆ Bring an extra dimension into your walk by silently repeating affirmations. Something like 'Every step brings me nearer to peace and contentment' or 'I'm in control of my life and at one with the world'.
◆ Walking is a good time to meditate.
◆ Buddhists practise a 'walking meditation' in which they move very slowly, noting every part of the movement. Feel the ground under your heel and the rest of your foot coming down to join it. You may lose your balance at first!
◆ When you're with children go at their pace, as the Chinese do. Stop to look at what interests them. It may take a little longer – though children are hard to rush anyway. But you'll arrive unstressed and, who knows, you may have had a more interesting journey.

▽ *Pump your arms like a race-walker at times, then slow down to your usual pace.*

Belly Dance – Eastern Promise

Any woman built on more generous lines than a catwalk model owes a debt of gratitude to those long-ago Middle Eastern women who entertained each other, on boring evenings in the harem, with a spot of belly dancing. Thanks to Hollywood, we've all seen how dynamic our natural curves can be when backed with some Arabian Nights music and a chiffon veil.

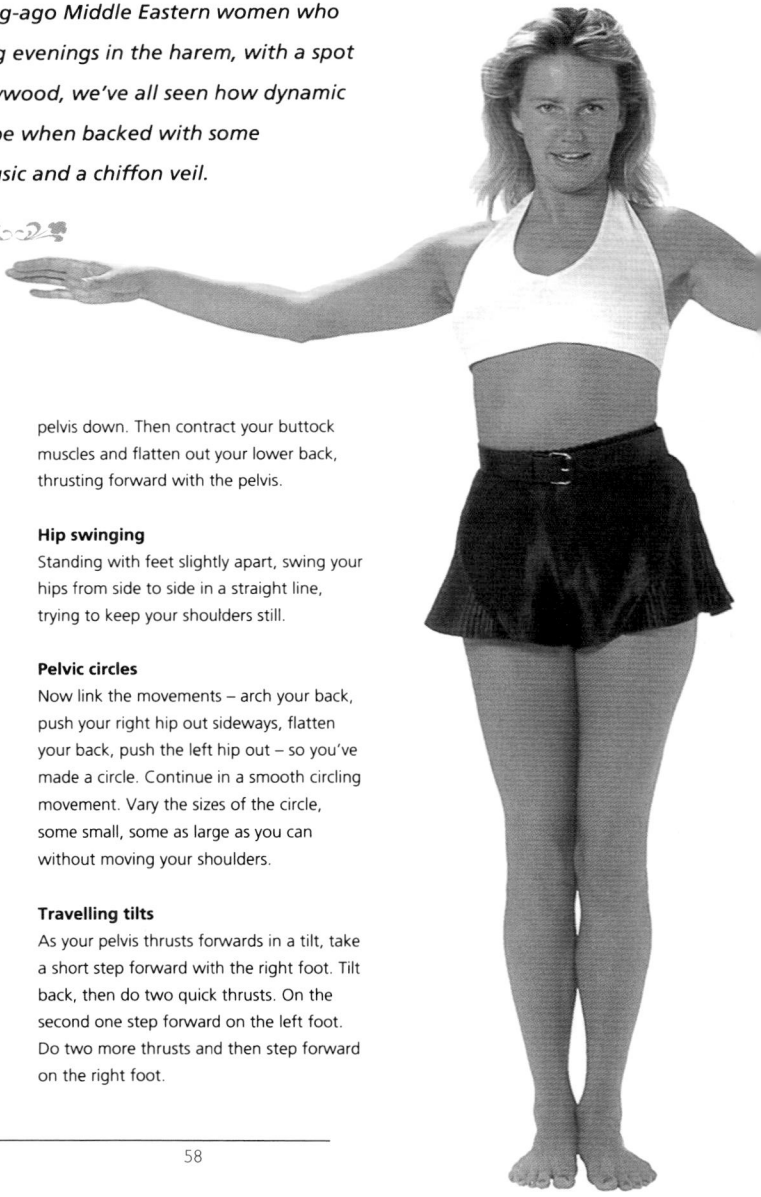

Belly dancing is such a fun form of exercise that you can now find classes in many towns, with costume-making and performances if you really get into it. Belly dancing includes something most of us never get – flexibility work. Our modern way of life limits us to a tiny range of movement leading inevitably to stiffness, lower back pain and aching joints.

In fact belly dance, or Raqs Sharqi, probably started as a symbolic enactment of giving birth and kept women in good shape for the real event. Its swaying movements ease aching muscles and, when the rhythm speeds up, it's an energizing aerobic workout.

Here are some basic moves, so treat yourself to a tape of Middle Eastern music and get shimmying. Navel-rubies optional!

Dancing from the centre

Practise each movement several times, then start linking them to create a smooth continuous dance.

Pelvic tilts

Stand with feet slightly apart, back straight, knees slightly bent. Arms should be by your side, slightly bent with palms facing forwards. Arch your back, tipping your pelvis down. Then contract your buttock muscles and flatten out your lower back, thrusting forward with the pelvis.

Hip swinging

Standing with feet slightly apart, swing your hips from side to side in a straight line, trying to keep your shoulders still.

Pelvic circles

Now link the movements – arch your back, push your right hip out sideways, flatten your back, push the left hip out – so you've made a circle. Continue in a smooth circling movement. Vary the sizes of the circle, some small, some as large as you can without moving your shoulders.

Travelling tilts

As your pelvis thrusts forwards in a tilt, take a short step forward with the right foot. Tilt back, then do two quick thrusts. On the second one step forward on the left foot. Do two more thrusts and then step forward on the right foot.

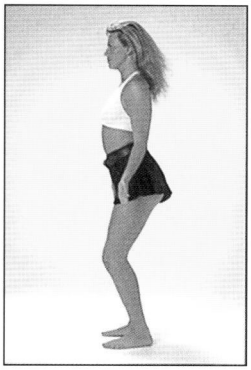

△ *From **travelling circles**...*

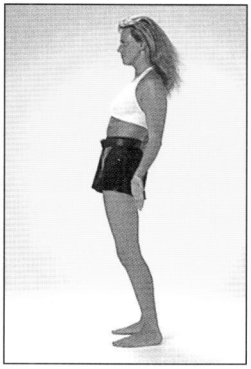

△ *Change to a **figure of eight**...*

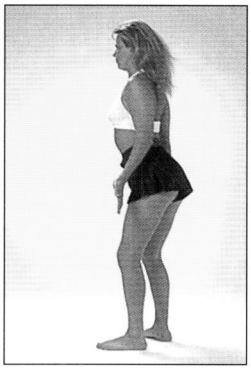

△ *Sideways in each direction...*

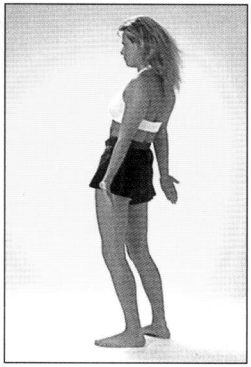

△ *It will take a bit of practice.*

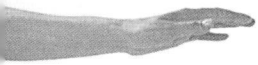

Travelling circles
As your hip comes round to the right take a small step forward with the right foot. Complete the circle, then as the hip moves left take a small step with the left foot. Remember to leave one and a half circles between steps.

Figure of eight
Next, change the circle to a figure of eight – sideways to the right, forward, back to the left, sideways to the left, forward, back to the right. It takes a bit of practice to create a smooth movement.

Belly roll
Suck your stomach in and lift your ribcage, so your back is slightly rounded. Then push your abdomen out, then in, in a continuous undulating movement.

Shimmy
With arms out beside you at shoulder level, move your shoulders backwards and forwards fast to shake your breasts.

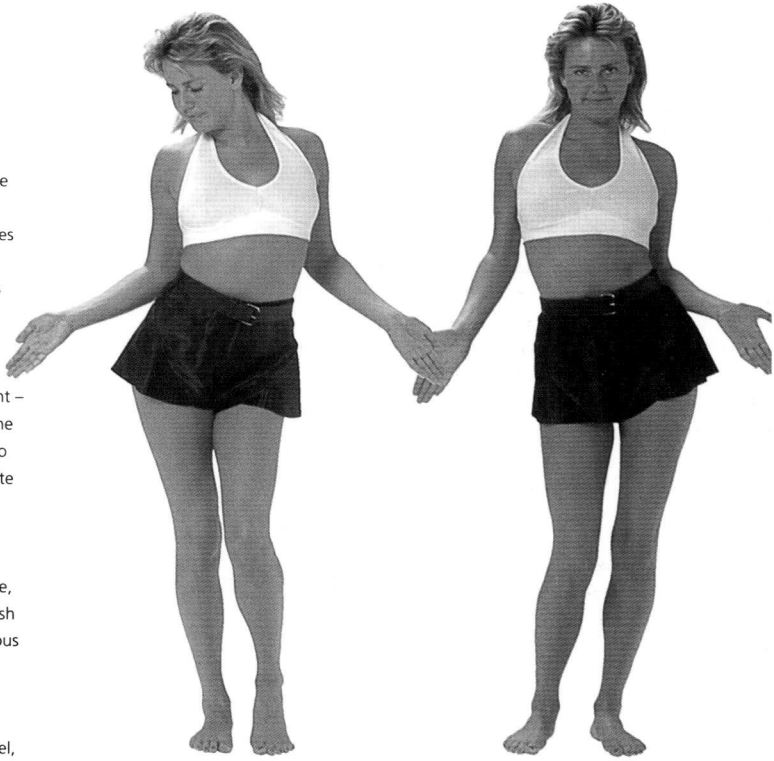

△ *Link the movements for pelvic tilts and hip swinging to create **pelvic circles**.*

△ *Vary the sizes of the circles, continuing without moving your shoulders.*

Autogenic Training

Harness Your Brain's Healing Powers

It sounds very technical, but in fact autogenic training is a simple way of teaching our bodies to relax. It's a down-to-earth technique, invented by a doctor in the 1920s, and is probably the most effective relaxation method developed by a westerner. But it has surprising effects – you can actually learn to make your skin warmer or cooler at will.

UNDER STRESS?

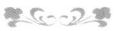

Autogenic training involves a series of mental exercises, telling yourself for example that your abdomen is warm and your forehead is cool. Eventually you will feel this healthy change in temperature – it has even been known to cure migraines. Like the other techniques in this book, it's not magic or linked with anything supernatural. It's just learning to put our natural abilities to good use.

You can learn autogenic training in small groups, meeting once a week and practising at home for about two months, or from books. It takes a little will-power at first, as with anything that involves learning and repeating a technique, especially if you use a book rather than classes. But it's not at all difficult, and since you practise while sitting or lying down comfortably, you don't need a lot of energy to get started. It's also handy because you can do it at any time.

The real beauty of autogenic training is that you're programming yourself to relax at will. The idea is that, once you've drummed a suggestion like 'My head and shoulders are heavy' into your brain often enough, you'll only have to say it to feel the effect. Your muscles really will feel heavy and relaxed as they instantly let go of tension. Having put in the work at the beginning, you should then have instant relaxation on tap.

◆ Don't try autogenic training if you suffer from epilepsy, insulin-dependent diabetes or schizophrenia, or within three months after a heart attack. If you suffer from glaucoma, make sure your condition is monitored.

▷ *Don't put up with stress, train your body to relax with this simple technique and enjoy instant relaxation on tap.*

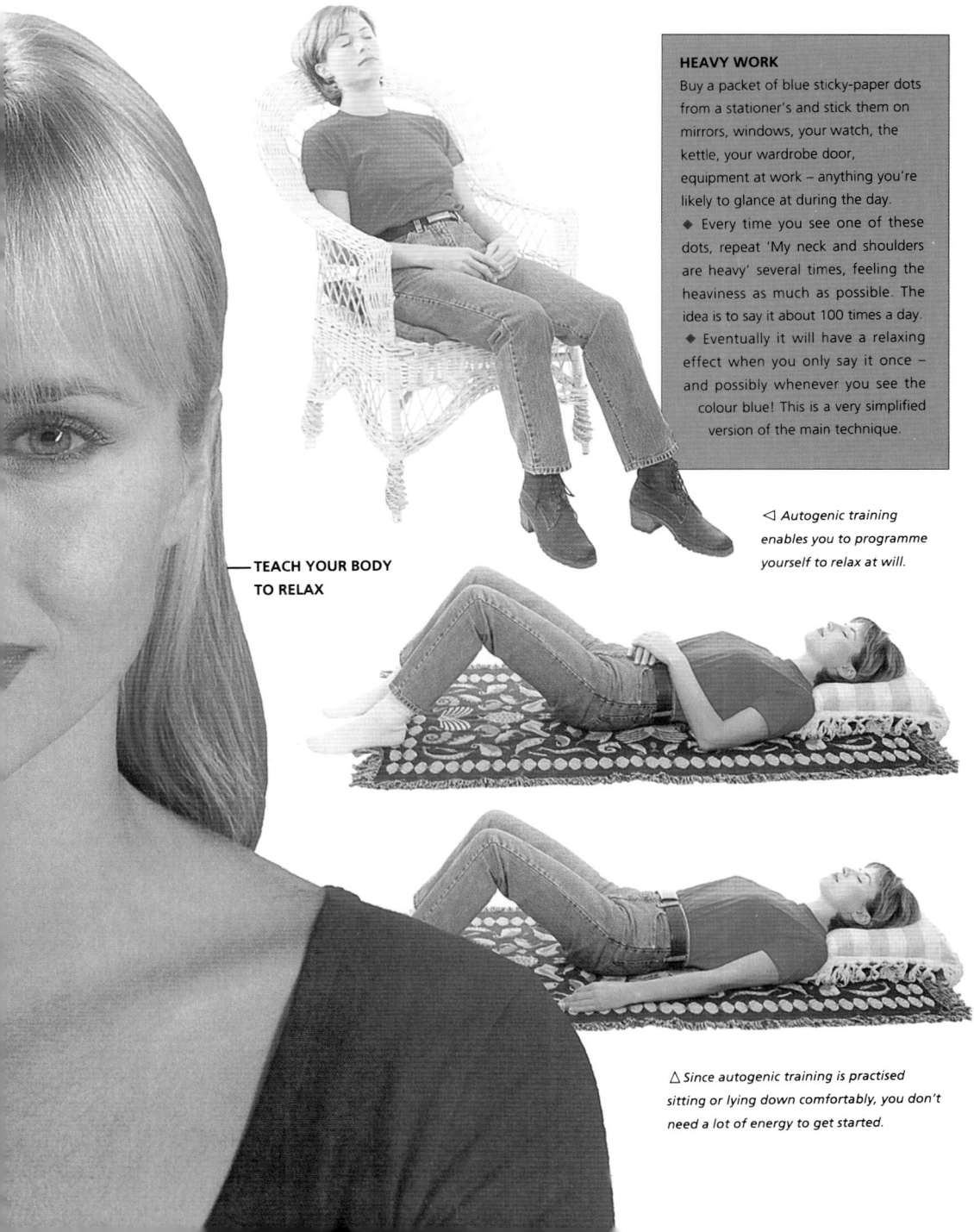

HEAVY WORK

Buy a packet of blue sticky-paper dots from a stationer's and stick them on mirrors, windows, your watch, the kettle, your wardrobe door, equipment at work – anything you're likely to glance at during the day.

◆ Every time you see one of these dots, repeat 'My neck and shoulders are heavy' several times, feeling the heaviness as much as possible. The idea is to say it about 100 times a day.

◆ Eventually it will have a relaxing effect when you only say it once – and possibly whenever you see the colour blue! This is a very simplified version of the main technique.

◁ Autogenic training enables you to programme yourself to relax at will.

TEACH YOUR BODY TO RELAX

△ Since autogenic training is practised sitting or lying down comfortably, you don't need a lot of energy to get started.

Meditation

Stilling The Mind's Chatter

If the word 'meditation' conjures up images of hippies and bearded gurus, think again. One of the most proven forms of stress relief, it's used by top business people and prescribed by doctors. The idea is to clear your mind by concentrating on one simple, even meaningless thing, such as counting. Then the brain switches from its busy everyday mode into the 'alpha' state – relaxed, alert and effective.

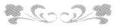

Meditation has been practised all over the world for thousands of years. Prayer, yoga, t'ai chi, breathing exercises, even the focusing methods that actors and athletes use – they're all forms of meditation. Think of stumbling though a toy-littered room with unwashed dishes cluttering every surface. Then see the same room clean, tidy and freshly painted. It's not a miracle, just a bit of work. Meditation has a similar effect on our minds.

You can learn it through religious and non-religious organizations, books and evening classes, including the expensive but effective Transcendental Meditation. Or simply use any of the following methods.

Seated meditation

Sit comfortably with your back straight. Set a timer for 10 minutes – eventually you can work up to 30 – and close your eyes. Let your thoughts subside and your breathing slow down. Stay focused on what you're doing. Don't breathe so deeply that you feel dizzy.

Counting

Count 'one' at the end of your first outbreath, 'two' at the end of the second, and so on. Start again from one when you reach 10 or if you drift off and lose your place.

Breath focus

Simply focus on the feel of the breath as it enters and leaves your nose. Alternatively, use any breathing exercises.

Mantra

Silently repeat a calming word or phrase with every outbreath, such as 'Peace', 'Stillness', 'Love', 'Joy', 'Yes', 'I am calm' or, if you have religious beliefs, 'God is love'. Try the Indian sacred word 'Om', which you can also say aloud on every outbreath.

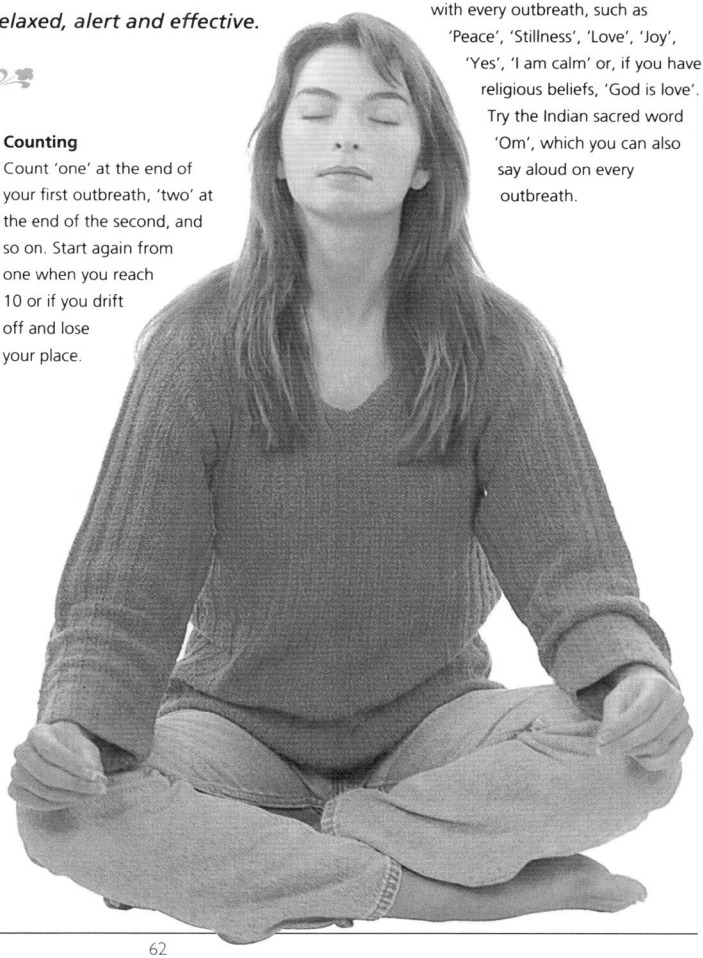

▷ *Sit comfortably with your back straight.*

Monkey-mind

Meditation stills the chatter that runs through our minds like a monkey swinging from branch to branch. But 'Monkey-mind' will put up a pretty good fight. It will produce endless distractions – anything to put off its bedtime! You just have to ignore it and keep bringing your attention back to meditating.

- Try to meditate at a set time and place every day.
- Choose one method and promise yourself you will do it every day for the next week.
- When thoughts come into your mind (as they do for everyone) just let them drift on out. Some people imagine wrapping them in a bubble and blowing them away. Calmly bring your mind back to the meditation.
- Very occasionally, meditation brings up a disturbing image. Just let it float out like any other – it's bubbled up like marsh gas and doesn't mean anything. If it bothers you, try a different technique such as mindfulness.
- Stick with it for the set time, even when it doesn't seem to be working. Meditation gets easier as you go on. And you get some benefit just from trying.

◁ *Clear your mind by counting or chanting.*

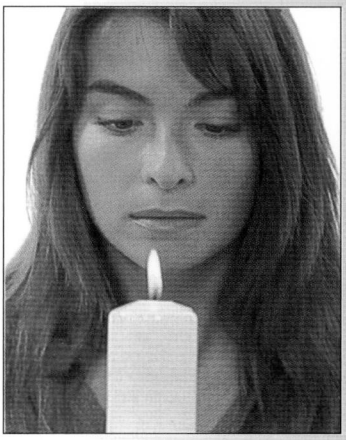

Candle

Instead of closing your eyes, light a candle and look at the flame, blinking as often as you need to.

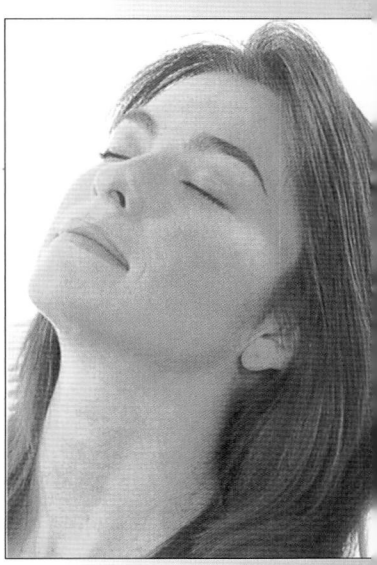

△ *Choose one method and promise you will do it each day for the next week. Try to meditate at the same time and in the same place every day.*

Mindfulness

Focusing on Where You Are

This has the same good effects as seated meditation but doesn't take up any time, because you practise it while you're doing other things. Mindfulness just means focusing on what you're doing – another way of quietening the mental chatter.

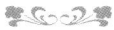

Most of the time we're only half aware of the present moment. Our minds run a constant background track of worries, daydreams, plans and memories. We mull over old arguments, giving ourselves a brilliant last word, and recall bits of last night's television. It's like a pile of junk mail in the head.

Because it's so distracting, this makes it hard to concentrate when we need to, and even when we're doing something for pleasure we're only half there.

Mindfulness is a way of training ourselves to be fully 'in the moment'. It makes work easier and good times more enjoyable. Then relaxation comes naturally.

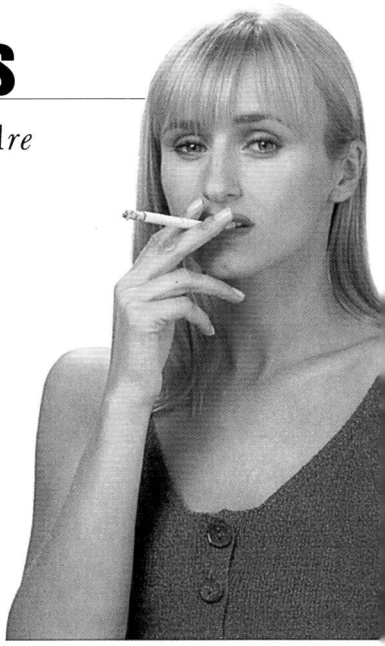

△ *Mindfulness techniques really do help people to give up smoking.*

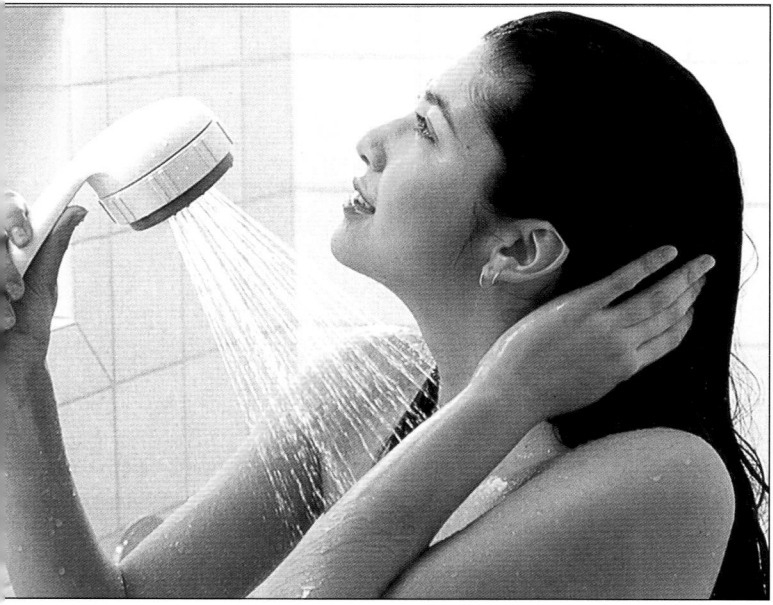

◁ *Practice mindfulness in the shower – be aware of the feel of the water on your skin.*

Mindfulness at work

- When you're washing up, instead of daydreaming or wondering what to get for the next meal, just be totally, calmly aware of what you're doing. Notice the feel of your hands slipping into warm water, the creamy texture of the bubbles, the sound of plates clinking against each other. Be aware of other sounds around you, but without thinking about them.
- The same with any other everyday chores and activities – we stop being like robots when we really experience the movement of a vacuum cleaner over a carpet, the speedy clicking of a keyboard, the swaying of a bus.

Smoke consciously to give up

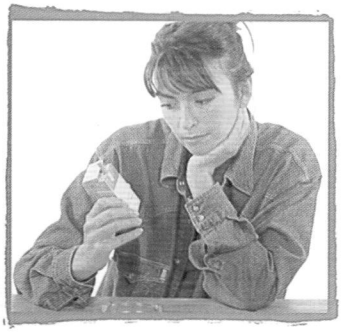

△ *Pick up the packet and really feel the shape and smoothness.*

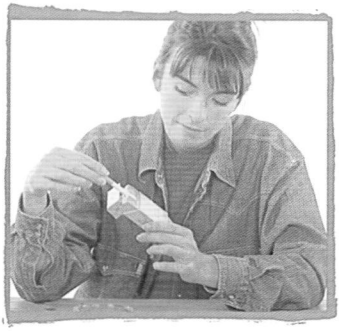

△ *Take out a cigarette and study it, focusing on the taste, smell and feel of it.*

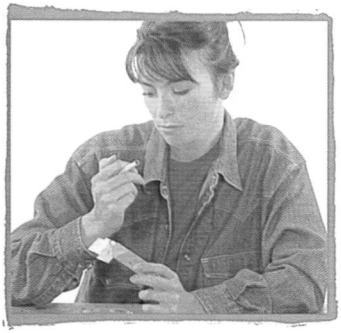

△ *Look at it as if you'd never seen a cigarette before.*

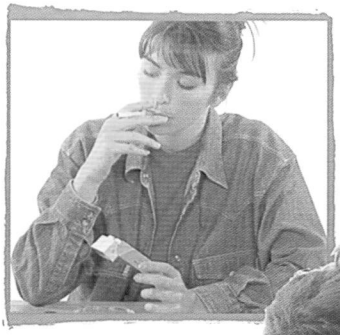

△ *Feel the cigarette in your hands and between your lips.*

▷ *Focus totally on it, right up until you slowly and mindfully stub it out.*

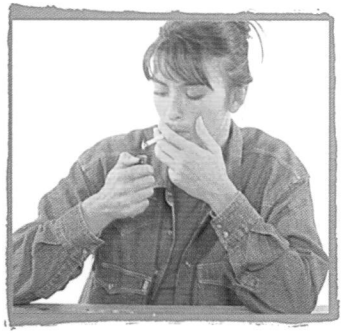

△ *Light the cigarette.*

◆ If you want to give up smoking, try smoking consciously. Pick up the packet. Hold it between both hands, really feeling the shape and smoothness. Take out a cigarette, look at it as if you'd never seen one before, feel it in your hands and between your lips. Don't smoke while you're doing anything else, but focus on the taste, smell and feel of it right up until you slowly and mindfully stub it out. Believe it or not, this has helped many people give up.

◆ Make sure you have time to sit down to a meal, then look at the food, smell it and notice how it makes you feel. Eat slowly and with pleasure, enjoying the texture as well as the taste, noting any memories or concerns that come to mind, but without dwelling on them.

The road to serenity

Mindfulness makes it easier to concentrate as well as preventing stress building up. After you've been practising for a while, so you're not distracted by doing things in this new frame of mind, try it when you are driving.

Keep your attention on all the things you need to do to drive safely, looking out for pedestrians and other traffic. Be aware of your own movements, your hands on the wheel, your feet on the pedals, instead of worrying about the time or other people's behaviour. Make this the best drive you are capable of.

Moving Meditation

Stillness in Action

If you find it hard to sit and meditate, why not try moving meditation? It's one step on from mindfulness – this time you're doing something active specifically to clear the mind.

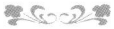

You can reach the relaxed, alert alpha state through all kinds of movement – dancing spontaneously or with learned steps (especially folk or circle dances), running, playing tennis. T'ai chi and yoga are forms of moving meditation.

It sometimes happens by itself when you're engrossed in an activity – when you feel the rhythm or music flowing through you as if you're part of it. You may even recognize it from times when you've been swimming or playing sports in the past.

When you're alone, try putting on some favourite music and dancing to it, not bothering about how you look but trying to follow the music, as if your body is becoming part of it. Dancing has a doubly stress-relieving effect, combining the relaxing benefits of moving and listening to music.

Experiment – try various different kinds of music, rap or classical or a folk tune – things you hadn't thought of dancing to. No need to try complicated steps. It's to let the music move your body and the movement still your mind.

Another route to moving meditation is through more formal exercise.

Energy moving

◆ Stand with back straight (not arched), arms by your sides. As you breathe in, raise your arms, palms up, stretching out to the fingertips as they reach above your head. Imagine yourself summoning up energy and breathing it in.

◆ On the outbreath turn the palms down and bring them slowly down beside you.

◆ Imagine breathing out your worries, and your hands bringing your stress levels down. Do this slowly at least 10 times and feel stress ebbing away.

Infinity

◆ Move your hips in the belly dance figure-of-eight (a horizontal eight, like this, is the symbol for infinity). Then let your body sway with it, arms circling at waist height like a Hawaiian dancer, and lose yourself in this timeless movement.

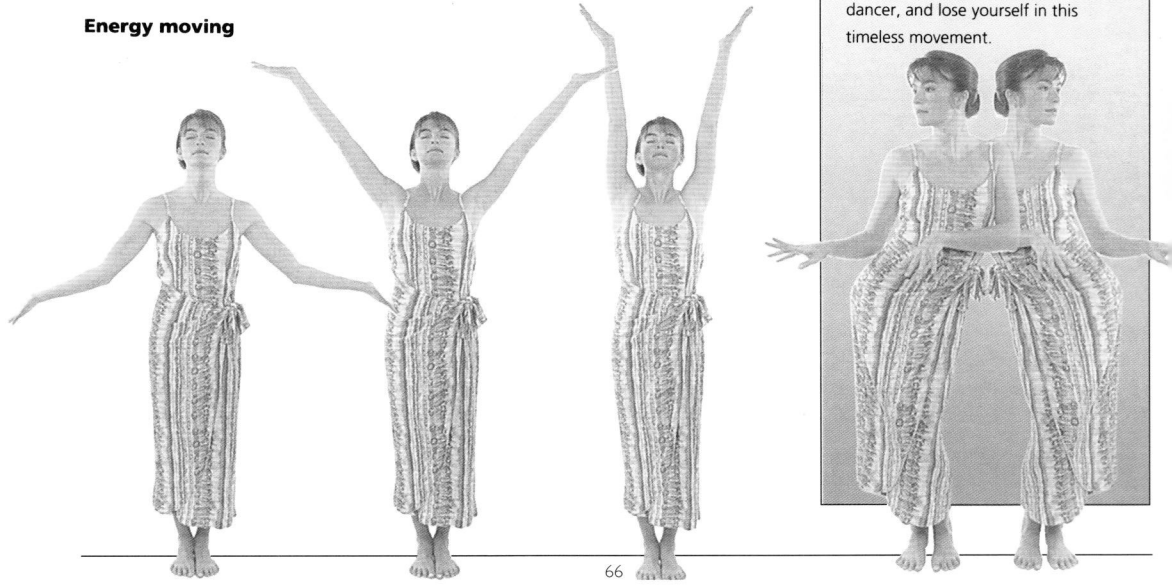

Water weed

◆ Put on music you could move to, without vocals. Stand with feet about shoulder-width apart, knees slightly bent, hands hanging loosely.

◆ Imagine you're a frond of water weed, being moved by tides and eddies. Let the water move your body in swirling motions including your arms and head, letting your knees bend.

◆ Flop forward from the waist and let the tide lift you up and round. Think of nothing but the water flowing around you.

Spiralling

◆ Sitting or kneeling with your back straight and head held high, breathe in and turn to the right, reaching out behind you with your right hand.

◆ Move from the hips, head and body moving as one. Stretch your arm back as far as it will comfortably go. Bring your outstretched arm up and reach for the ceiling as you face forward again.

◆ As you start breathing out, turn to the left and bring your arm down and across to the left thigh, in a smooth spiral motion.

◆ Keep breathing steadily as you repeat the movement with the left arm towards the right side.

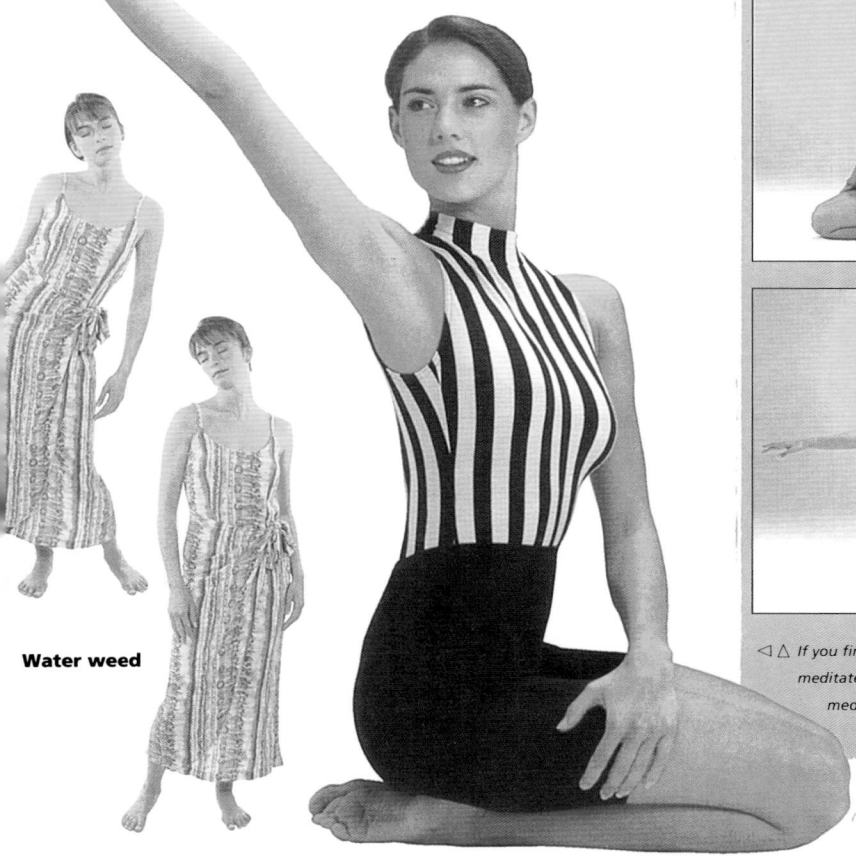

Water weed

Spiralling

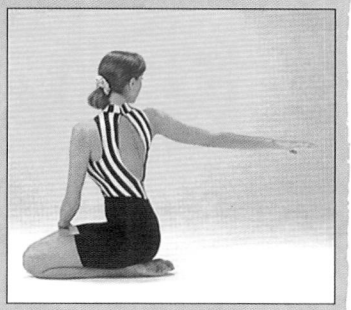

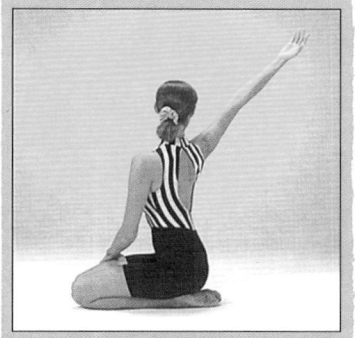

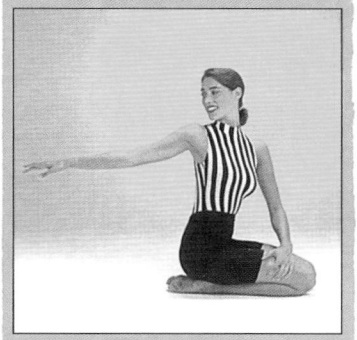

◁ △ *If you find it hard to sit still and meditate, clear your mind with moving meditation.*

Hypnosis – Reach Your Inner Self

Say 'hypnosis' and most people will think of a melodramatic villain with piercing eyes, or a stage full of revellers who all think they're Elvis. Yet its most popular use these days is in hypnotherapy – a way of solving problems through the power of the patient's own mind.

Hypnotherapists are setting up shop all over the country, and – judging from the number of people who say they've been helped to relax, lose their phobias, control panic attacks or give up smoking – it can do a lot of good.

Being hypnotized is quite a relaxing experience in itself, but that's not its main point. It's a way of bypassing the conscious mind so the therapist can implant helpful suggestions such as 'I am perfectly relaxed' or 'I easily do all my work and still have plenty of energy' in the subconscious, which accepts them more readily.

Why bypass the conscious mind? Because it's full of everyday clutter and worries. If you say 'I am relaxed' it's just as likely to retort 'No you're not, or you wouldn't be doing this'.

Some hypnotherapists also offer psychotherapy – which may include discovering how events from the past still cause tension in your life, and how to get them out of your system. It's easier to do while you're in a relaxed state.

Seeing a hypnotherapist

At your first visit the hypnotherapist is likely to ask a few questions about your health and why you've come. You'll sit in a comfortable chair or lie down with your eyes closed, while the hypnotherapist talks you through a relaxation routine

▽ *Being hypnotised can be very relaxing.*

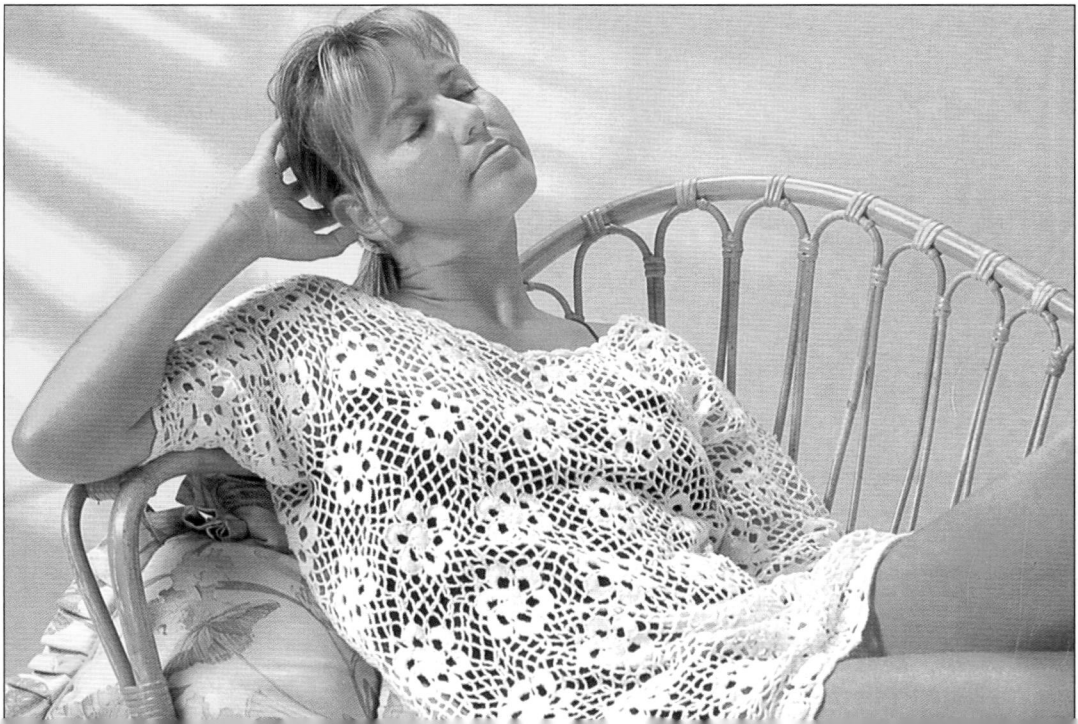

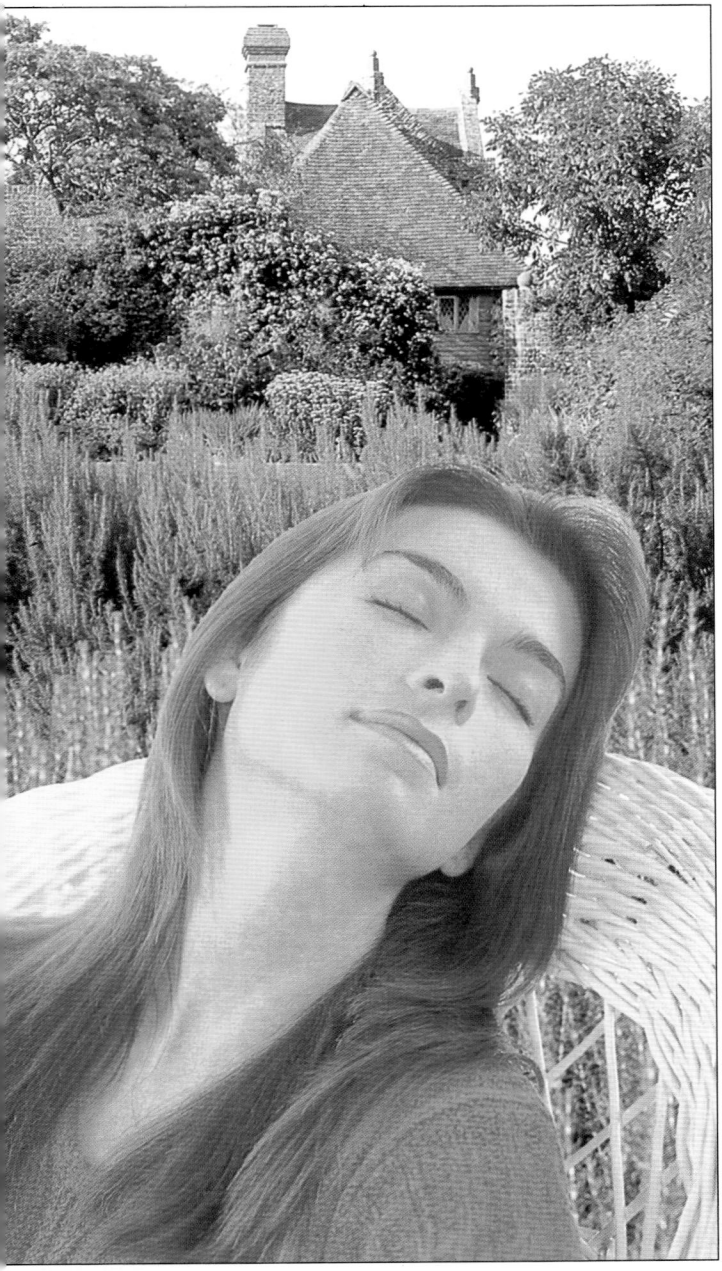

or invites you to imagine you're in a beautiful, peaceful place. It's not a hands-on therapy, though she may lift your arm to check if the muscles are relaxed.

Once you're deeply relaxed she'll make suggestions like 'I feel comfortable in all social situations', or whatever is relevant, and may teach you a phrase or simple technique to bring back that calm state of mind when you do it in future.

You remain conscious the whole time, probably feeling quite dreamy and very relaxed. When the therapist asks you to come out of the trance you do so at once – possibly not realising you've actually been under hypnosis!

Many hypnotherapists will give instructions on self-hypnosis to take home, and you may only need the one session.

WHAT COULD GO WRONG?

◆ Hypnosis can't make you do something you'd consider totally wrong or dangerous. You might be persuaded to cluck like a chicken but not to stab someone. In rare cases male hypnotherapists have taken advantage of a client's relaxed and suggestible state, but that's abuse of trust, not mystic powers.

◆ Unlike a stage hypnotist, a properly trained hypnotherapist can make sure you're fully back to everyday consciousness before you leave.

◆ Any form of psychotherapy, with or without hypnosis, may bring up a lot of distress. So don't start unless you can afford as many sessions as it takes to sort out – and then only with someone you're sure is trustworthy and has the right professional skills. A family doctor can often make recommendations.

◁ *Imagine you're in a beautiful place.*

Self-Hypnosis

Give Yourself Some Useful New Instructions

You can hypnotize yourself if you put your mind to it. It's not dangerous – you can't get 'stuck' under hypnosis or give yourself some harmful command. You'll just use the space given by deep relaxation to put some constructive thoughts where they'll do most good.

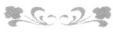

Start by lying on the floor or sitting in a straight-backed chair, hands in your lap. If you have time, go through the foot-to-head relaxation. If time is short, do some breathing exercises to set the scene and put you in a calm and peaceful frame of mind.

Getting started

- You can do this without making a tape, but it's easier to follow spoken instructions – simply read out the script on this page.

  Speak in a slow, calm, rather monotonous voice and remember to leave pauses. You can give yourself any suggestions you like on your secluded beach, but they must be positive, clear and harmless.
- In an emergency, just say to yourself, 'One, two three, ready.' You can snap out of hypnosis instantly, but a brief wake-up formula reduces the jolt.
- If you find it hard to visualize, just do the counting – many people find this equally effective.
- For deeper relaxation use 30 steps down to the beach instead of 10.

The script

Say to yourself, 'Everything I am doing makes me healthier, more relaxed, and more in control of my life. I will wake up immediately if I need to.'

When you feel comfortably relaxed, imagine sitting on a wooden bench in a beautiful garden, full of flowers. Bees are buzzing gently, and the sun warms your skin. At the end of the garden there's a gate. You walk through, noting the rough texture of the weathered wood as you push it open.

Beyond it are steps leading down to a secluded beach, with waves gently lapping on the sand. You walk slowly down, feeling the coolness of stone under your feet as you count the steps – one, two, three... at every step you feel more relaxed... four, five, six... deeply calm and relaxed... seven, eight, nine... your body is relaxed, your mind open to all the good that can come to you here... 10.

You are on this beautiful beach, knowing you are perfectly safe and can leave whenever you want. Enjoy the peace and serenity. Nearby you see a wrought-iron seat facing the sea. You sit down and say to yourself, 'I am peaceful, happy and perfectly in control of my life. I easily cope with everything that happens.'

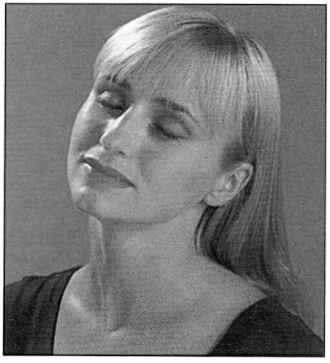

△ *You are on a beautiful beach, with waves gently lapping on the sand... you are perfectly safe and can return whenever you want.*

Now pinch the fold of skin between thumb and first finger on your right hand (pinch your thumb if you're pregnant). From now on you can relax at will, simply by doing that and remembering this peaceful place.

Repeat, 'I am peaceful, happy and perfectly in control of my life. I easily cope with everything that happens. I can relax at will, simply by pinching my right hand and thinking of this place.'

When you're ready, return to the steps, knowing you can come back here any time you like. You will return to everyday consciousness as you count down, but will be able to relax at will. Count slowly down from 10, as you walk up the steps, starting to notice the everyday sounds around you. By zero you are back to everyday consciousness, relaxed and alert.

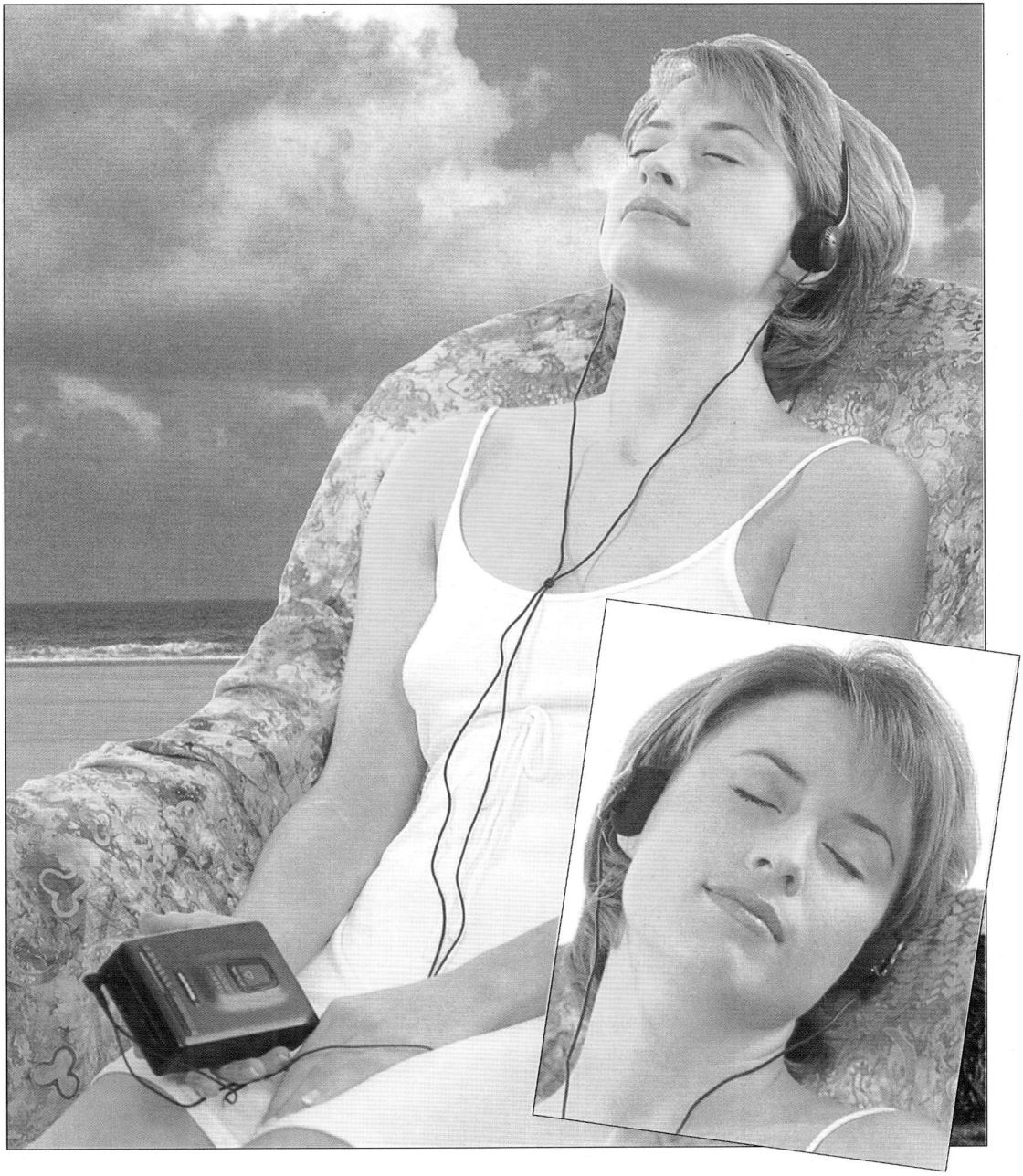

Colour Therapy

The Shades That Change Your Moods

Next time you see red, think blue – it's such a calming colour that even the thought of it brings raised blood pressure down. Colours affect us more than we may think – warm ones like red, pink, orange and yellow are stimulating, while the cool hues – green, blue, turquoise and violet – are calming. Blue is generally considered most relaxing. Green promotes balance, as does dignified violet. Turquoise is refreshing and calming.

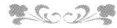

Our choice of clothes both reflects and reinforces our feelings – flamboyant, outgoing colours, quiet neutrals, the dark shades of sadness, bold patterns, big cheerful flowers.

For a change, try wearing blue, green or violet – as pure and clear as possible – when you need to feel more relaxed, balanced or confident. It doesn't have to be head to foot – a bright silk scarf will do. If the pure colour doesn't suit you try a different shade, or wear it as trousers or a skirt.

The same at home – choose tranquil colours for the bathroom and bedroom. A picture of blue sky and green countryside is deeply soothing. Remember, though, that walls painted in any strong colour may be overwhelming and cold blues can be depressing. You can use the chosen colour as a highlight in bedding, towels, coloured bath oils, curtains, cushions, wallpaper patterns or anything you like to look at. White paint with a hint of colour continues the theme in an unobtrusive background.

Don't ban warm colours though, or your home could have a chilly feel. Pink and peachy shades are comforting. An all-red room would be oppressive, but it's a revitalising colour and touches of red perk the place up.

Oh, and don't worry if teenagers shroud themselves in black, says colour therapist Susan Farrar, it's a kind of cocoon – they're coping with the death of childhood and absorbing major changes. Who knows what butterflies will emerge?

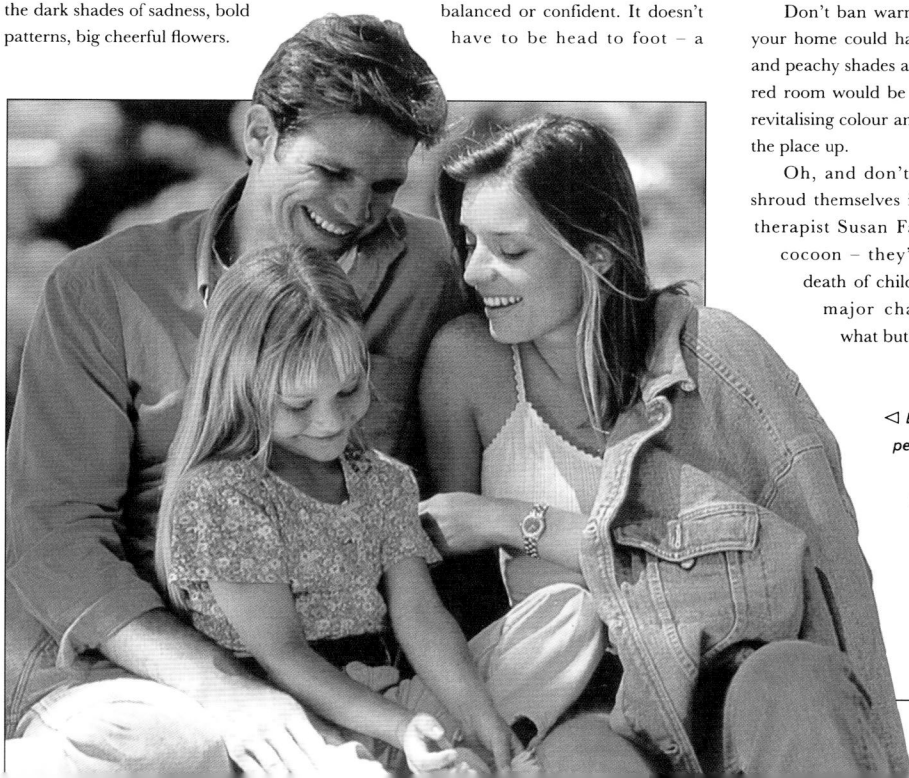

◁ Blue is the colour of peace and tranquillity.

▷ To restore balance, breathe fully into your abdomen at a natural pace. Breathe in green – breathe out magenta.

Colour breathing

◆ For happiness and fun imagine breathing in the colour orange – breathe out blue.
◆ Violet increases self-respect – breathe out yellow.
◆ Breathe in yellow when you need to feel some detachment from things – breathe out violet.
◆ Green cleanses and balances – breathe out magenta.
◆ Breathe in magenta to let go of obsessional thoughts – breathe out green.
◆ Red is for vitality – breathe out turquoise.
◆ Turquoise strengthens the immune system – breathe out red.

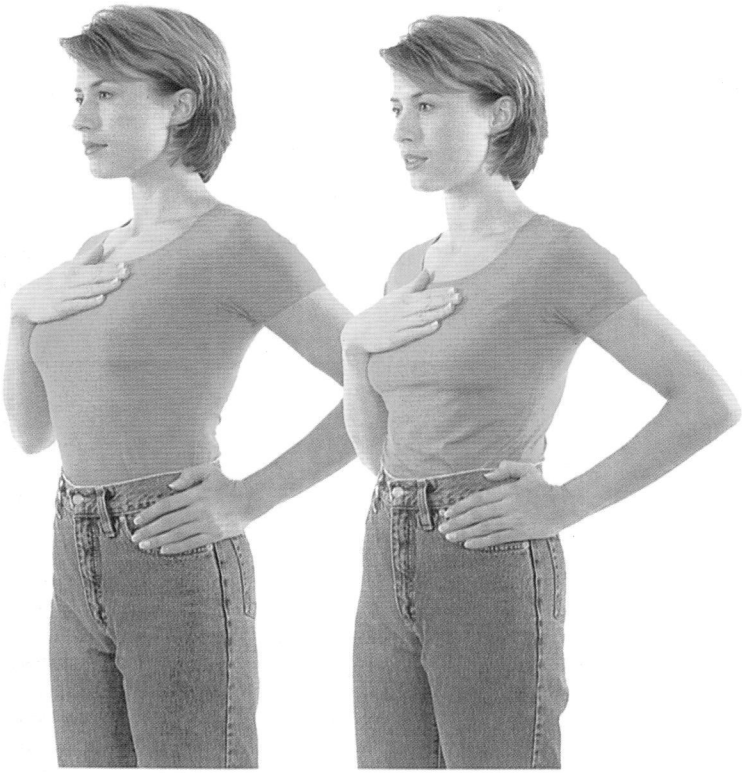

Colour visualization

Theo Gimbel recommends the effective exercises on this page in his *Book of Colour Healing*, using complementary colours for balance and well-being.

◆ Start by relaxing your muscles, for example with the foot-to-head technique.
◆ Then lie or sit comfortably with your back straight, eyes closed, and think of yourself at a time when you were particularly well and happy.
◆ Keep this positive image in mind and let other thoughts drift away.
◆ Breathe fully into your abdomen, at a natural pace.
◆ As you breathe in, imagine sitting by a blue lake under a calm blue sky.
◆ Feel the calmness of the blue fill your body.
◆ On the outbreath, imagine you are looking at the intense orange of a marigold.
◆ Repeat this several times, then sit quietly for a while.
◆ You can also imagine the colour blue entering your solar plexus (just below the chest) as you breathe in, and spreading around your body beneath the skin.
◆ Imagine breathing out the colour orange.

Voice & Music Therapy

Sound Advice

Stress tightens our throats (ever heard your voice come out in a squeak when you were nervous?) and, in the long term, restricts breathing without our even noticing. Using your voice not only loosens the throat – the vibration is said to benefit the whole body, like an internal massage.

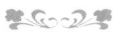

Singing is a wonderful way to relax. Oh I know, most of us are convinced we squawk like crows. But voice teachers retort, 'If you can talk you can sing,' and they're right. You may not sound like an operatic diva – but no one says that you're not allowed to run if you're below Olympic standard.

All over the world people sing to express their feelings – joy, grief, anger, spirituality, love and longing. Giving up this simple, universal pleasure is like losing the right to dance or play. No wonder so many of us suffer from tense facial muscles, causing headaches and premature wrinkles.

So let your voice dance. Sing in your bath, while you're working, with the radio, in the car or with small children – they love it. Sing scales or make up tunes with the sound 'aaa' or 'oh'.

Don't worry if your voice sounds tight or quavery, weak or rusty – imagine what your leg muscles would be like if you hadn't used them since childhood. You'll be surprised how quickly it grows confident and strong.

The yoga lion

- Loosen up by sitting comfortably, with palms resting on your lap.
- As you breathe out, open your mouth and eyes wide and slowly stick your tongue out as far as possible.
- Splay out your fingers and look fierce, then relax as you breathe in.
- Repeat several times.

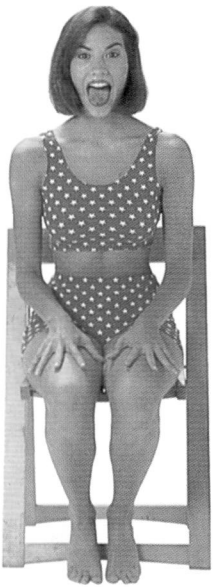

▷ *The yoga lion is a great exercise to loosen up those neglected facial muscles!*

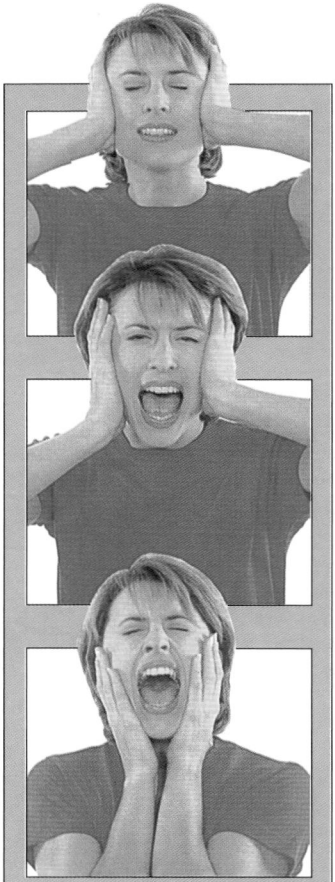

Letting It Out

Screaming is a great stress-reliever. It eases tension around the face as well as relieving pent-up feelings. At night, try it in the car with windows closed. But the best place for screaming is a funfair – choose a scary ride and shriek to your heart's content.

Reclaim your voice

Find a quiet spot where you won't worry about being overheard, then try some of these exercises, suggested by voice therapists Susan Lever and Frankie Armstrong. Don't strain to reach a note, your range will expand naturally.

- If you're tired, do some huge, exaggerated yawns to release tension around the mouth.
- If you're stressed and irritable, give some long and noisy sighs. Progress to deep groans if you feel like it.
- Humming has a soothing effect as it resonates through your body. Notice where you feel it and if it changes when you alter the note.
- Exaggerate some everyday sounds, taking a deep breath and seeing how long and varied you can make them on the outbreath. Say 'Oh!' as if you'd just heard a thrilling piece of gossip, starting at a normal level and sending your voice as high and then as low as it will go. Try a baffled 'Eh?' sending your voice up to the top of its pitch. Then a grumpy 'Huh', letting all the breath out in a long growly 'hhhh'. What about an 'Mmmm' going up and down the scale? And a deliciously scandalized 'Ooooh!'
- Sing pure vowel sounds on one long, strong note:
  'ah' as in 'past'
  'e' as in 'went'
  'ee' as in 'piece'
  'o' as in 'on'
  'oo' as in 'flute'.

This can have the same effect on brainwaves as meditating.

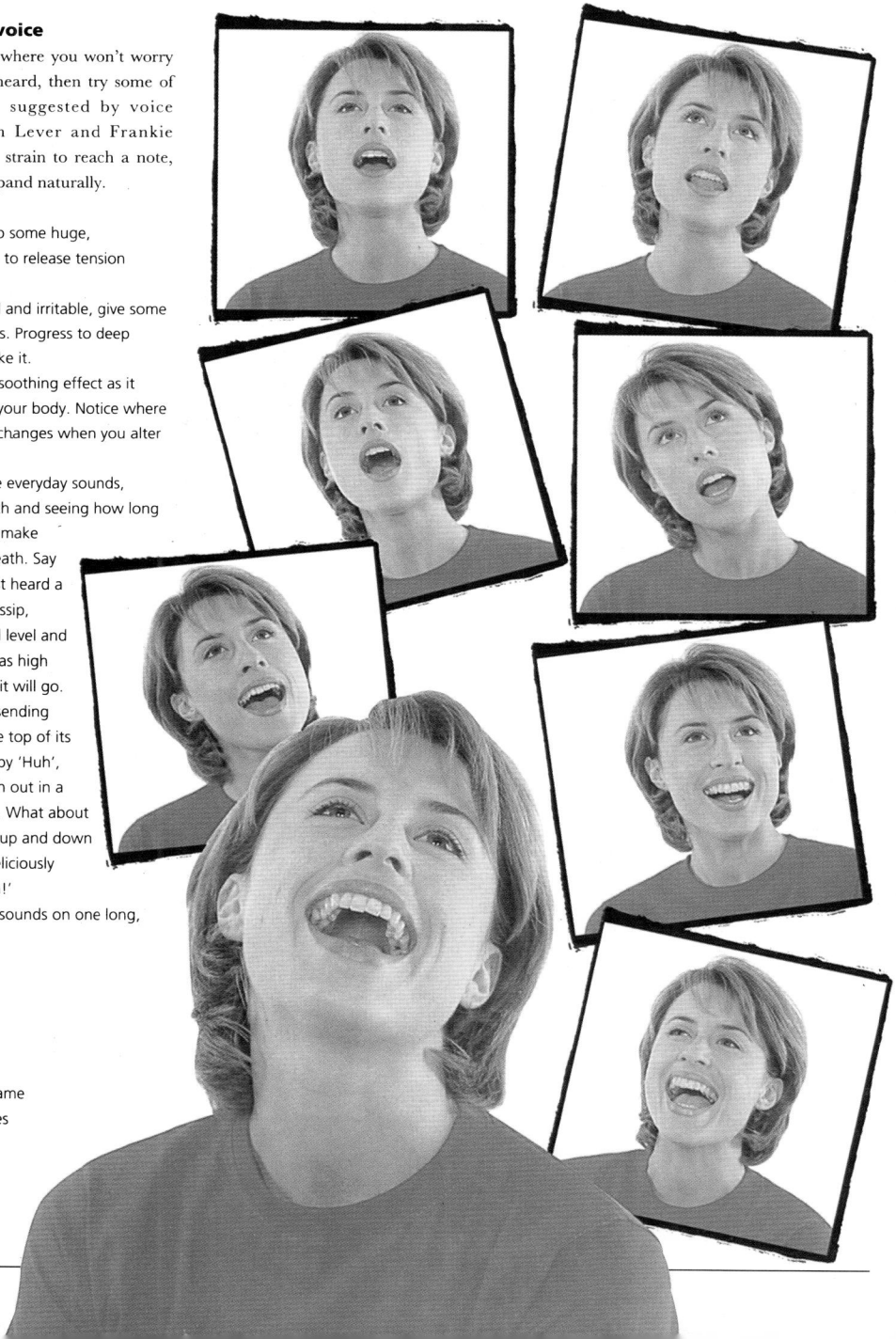

Herbalism – Power of Plants

Long before scientists thought of creating drugs from plants, our ancestors used the whole plants to make a more balanced remedy. Today, a stroll through any health food shop will once again reveal herbal potions aimed at relieving stress. Where tranquillizers act like a blow with a blunt object, these have a gentler soothing effect to help the body through crises.

A handful of relaxing herbs tied in a cloth and hung under the hot tap makes a special bath after a hectic day.

The most popular way of taking herbal remedies, though, is as a cup of tea. Simplest of all are the many different herbal teabags now available, even in supermarkets. Look out for those produced organically, without any agricultural chemicals, and experiment to find your favourite flavours.

Some herbs have a medicinal tang and valerian has even been likened to smelly socks. But others are only lightly scented and some, like camomile and peppermint, seem to please most tastes.

◁ Brew up a cup of soothing herbal tea with the fragrance of camomile or the refreshing tang of lemon balm.

Growing your own

Fresh air, exercise, useful work and feeling at one with nature – no wonder so many people love gardening. Even with a few pots on a windowsill, you can create a herb garden to supply you all year round, freshly picked or harvested at the right time of year and hung up to dry.

Mint, for example, grows like a weed and is often planted in containers to stop it taking over the entire garden. Skullcap, lavender, valerian, lemon balm – none of them need a green-fingered gardener. And, unlike growing flowers or veg, you can produce a useful and lovely-smelling herb garden with very little work.

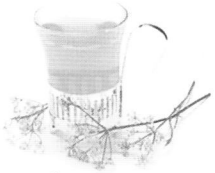

Playing safe

'Natural' doesn't mean weak or harmless. In China, where traditional medicine is still taught at medical school level, herbalists prescribe concoctions with wonderdrug-like effects.

Even in Europe – where much of the herbal lore was lost after its users were branded as witches – modern practitioners have produced some startling cures. That kind of powerful brew is best made by qualified practitioners.

All the herbs recommended here can be made into a tea or 'infusion', by pouring hot water onto a teaspoonful or two and letting it brew in a teapot till it's cool enough to strain and drink.

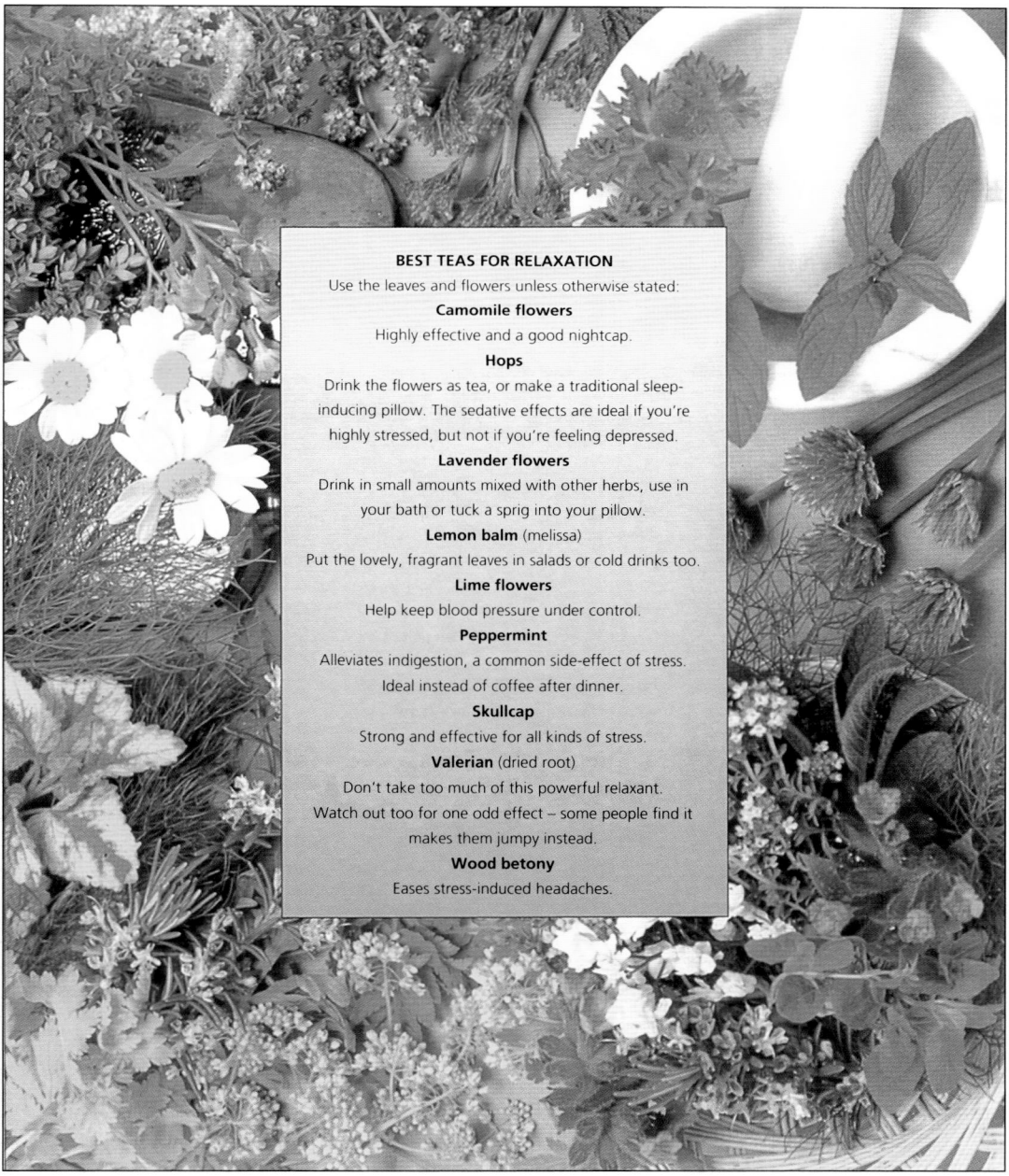

BEST TEAS FOR RELAXATION

Use the leaves and flowers unless otherwise stated:

Camomile flowers

Highly effective and a good nightcap.

Hops

Drink the flowers as tea, or make a traditional sleep-inducing pillow. The sedative effects are ideal if you're highly stressed, but not if you're feeling depressed.

Lavender flowers

Drink in small amounts mixed with other herbs, use in your bath or tuck a sprig into your pillow.

Lemon balm (melissa)

Put the lovely, fragrant leaves in salads or cold drinks too.

Lime flowers

Help keep blood pressure under control.

Peppermint

Alleviates indigestion, a common side-effect of stress. Ideal instead of coffee after dinner.

Skullcap

Strong and effective for all kinds of stress.

Valerian (dried root)

Don't take too much of this powerful relaxant. Watch out too for one odd effect – some people find it makes them jumpy instead.

Wood betony

Eases stress-induced headaches.

Homeopathy – Like Cures Like

Homeopathy has been in use for 200 years, longer than most drugs. It has always been available on Britain's National Health Service and the royal family's doctor is a homeopath. But homeopathy runs on totally different principles from orthodox medicine.

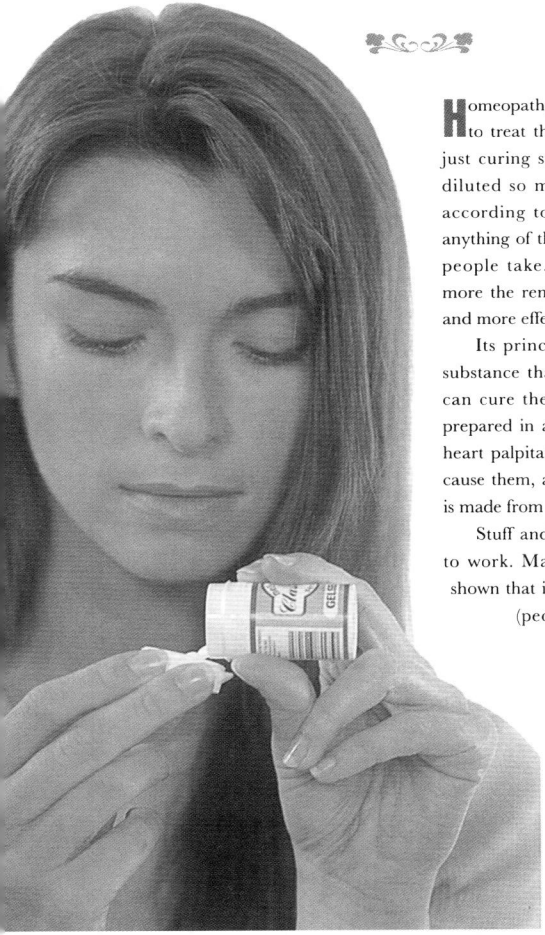

Homeopathy is holistic, meaning it aims to treat the whole person rather than just curing symptoms. Its remedies are diluted so many thousand times that, according to scientists, there can't be anything of them left in the pills or drops people take. Yet homeopaths say the more the remedy is diluted, the stronger and more effective it becomes.

Its principle is 'like cures like' – a substance that causes certain symptoms can cure them if used in tiny amounts prepared in a certain way. A remedy for heart palpitations uses coffee, which can cause them, and the cure for insect stings is made from bees.

Stuff and nonsense? Oddly, it seems to work. Many reputable studies have shown that it's not just the placebo effect (people getting better because they think they will), it often has better results than conventional medicines, even when used for the treatment of animals.

◁ *To keep the remedy in its purest form, don't let it touch anything, even your fingers.*

◆ Tip tablets into the bottle top, then straight into your mouth without handling them.

◆ Don't eat, drink, smoke or brush your teeth for at least 15 minutes before and after taking a remedy.

Each remedy also suits a different type of person. So if you have a long-standing health problem, a homeopath will work out which of the homeopathic types you are and prescribe that remedy – to treat you rather than the disease.

For example, are you worried about a forthcoming event such as an exam? Do you set yourself high standards and fear you won't reach them? Do you crave sweet foods? Do you lie awake fretting about the past day? Do you feel better after midnight, when moving around, in cool surroundings, or after hot food or drinks? Do you feel worse in stuffy atmospheres, in the early evening and if you overeat? If so, you're a Lycopodium clavatum person! Few of us fit such a detailed picture, of course, but if most of it sounds like you that remedy could put you right.

Don't be put off trying for yourself. The more honest you can be about your character, the easier it will be to diagnose yourself from a book. And some remedies have more general first-aid uses.

▷ *Main picture, right: Bluebell (Agraphis nutans). Small pictures from left: Common daisy (Bellis perennis); foxglove (Digitalis purpurea); St John's wort (Hypericum perforatum); blue flag (Iris versicolor).*

DO-IT-YOURSELF REMEDIES

Aconitum napellus, a first resort for fear or panic attacks and after physical trauma.

Anacardium for anxiety caused by indecisiveness, possibly hidden under a tough exterior.

Argentum nitricum when you're so worried you can't concentrate.

Arnica for emotional or physical shock.

Arsenicum album for anxiety in a perfectionist.

Avena sativa for exhaustion caused by long-term anxiety.

Carbo vegetabilis for shock causing clammy hands.

Coffea for insomnia caused by an overactive mind – or too much coffee.

Colocynthis for anger that causes headaches or indigestion.

Gelsemium for shock, or worry that's making you feel irritable and tearful.

Ignatia amara for shock, where you're trying unsuccessfully to stay in control.

Kali phosphoricum for jaded nerves.

Stramonium for a bout of sudden, intense panic.

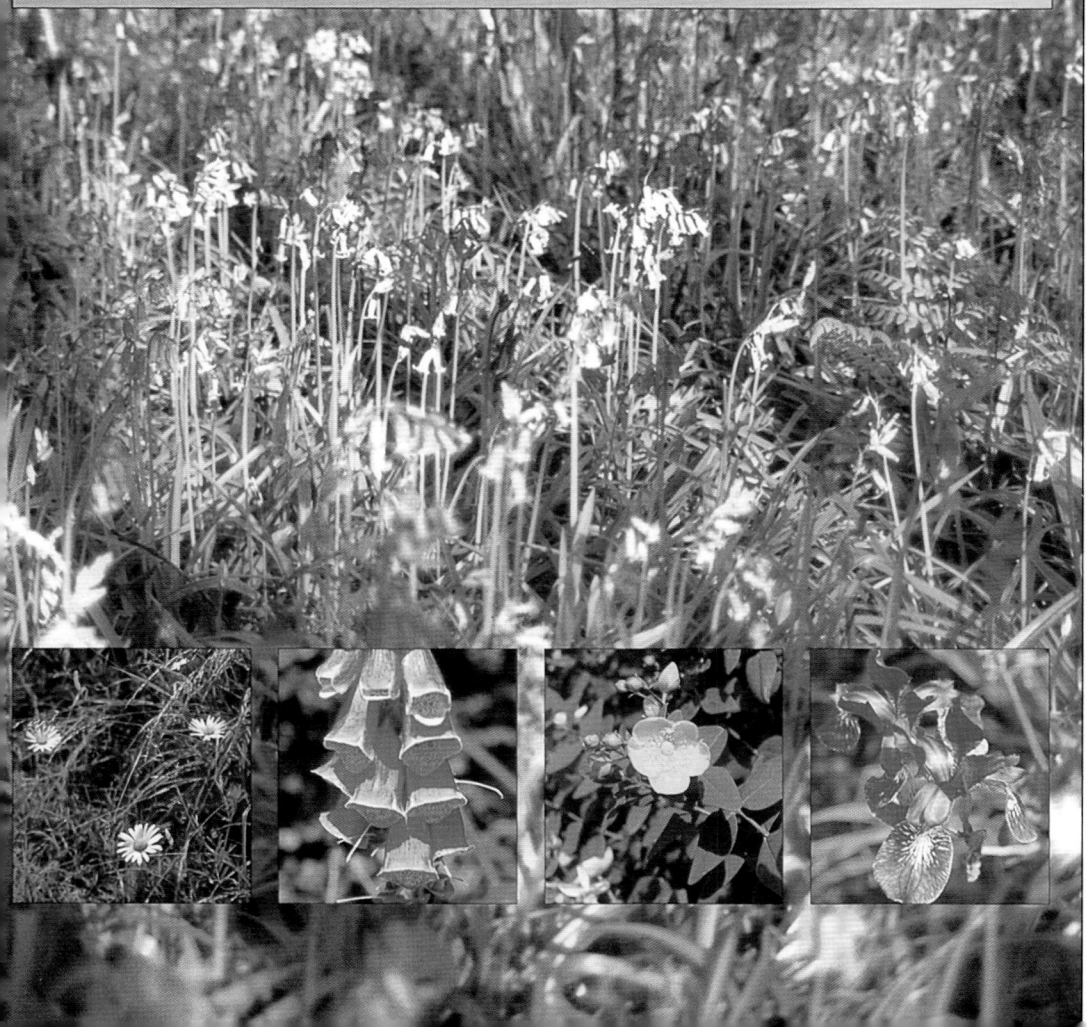

Flower Remedies

Subtly Working on Emotions

Even gentler than homeopathy, flower remedies aim to combat stress and illness by balancing our emotional energies. It's easy to see why people should think flowers can heal psychological wounds. Their delicate beauty and fragrance have always been linked with spirituality.

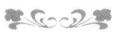

In the 1930s, idealistic homeopath Dr Edward Bach (pronounced 'batch') came to believe flowers have an affinity with the human soul and could put people back in tune with their higher natures. This in turn would reduce illness, which is so often caused by mental stresses.

He developed a range of 38 essences, which he believed dealt with every emotional state people could suffer.

The remedies aren't claimed to solve problems directly – how could they? – but are aimed at helping people bring their feelings back into balance.

Since then other practitioners around the world have taken up the idea and there are now about two dozen different ranges containing more than

◁ *Flower remedies can be taken simply by putting a few drops on or under the tongue.*

FROM AROUND THE WORLD

Look out for some of the many different ranges now on offer. Several also include emergency remedies.

◆ Australian Bush Flower Essences include waratah to help deal with stress and use our survival skills, mountain devil for high blood pressure, jacaranda for nervousness and black-eyed Susan for hyperactivity.

◆ From Findhorn in Scotland come Scottish primrose for peace, broom for clarity of mind and thistle for courage.

◆ Himalayan Indian Tree and Flower Essences include pongham tree to rest the brain, commelina to calm the nerves and red-hot cat tail to prevent over-impulsiveness.

◆ From Andreas Korte's African and Amazon range; cinnamon rose to restore hope, dandelion for reducing tension and wild carrot to stop thoughts racing around the brain.

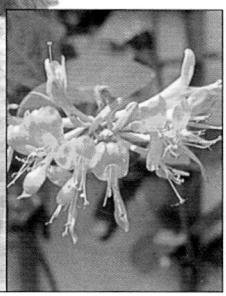

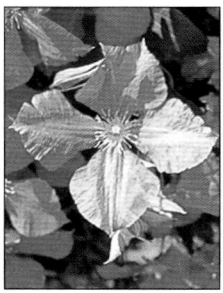

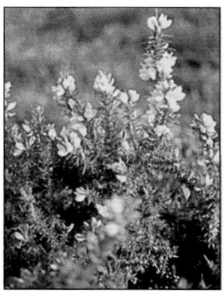

△ *From left: Honeysuckle for living in the past, clematis for lack of interest and gorse for despair.*

1,200 remedies. That's everything from New Zealand's abelia, which helps balance our rational and emotional sides, to the African zinnia, which helps us loosen up and re-learn how to laugh. Some cover aspects Bach didn't deal with, including sexuality.

Bach remedies seem to be the easiest to find – the little bottles are widely sold in pharmacies and health food shops. You can use up to half a dozen at a time, putting a few drops in a drink or straight onto your tongue. Rescue Remedy is the best known – a blend of impatiens, star of Bethlehem, cherry plum, rock rose and clematis to relieve stress and panic in an emergency.

Some remedies contain alcohol as a preservative, but they're all harmless and can be used alongside any medical treatment.

▷ *Wild rose, used to treat apathy.*

▽ *At least one of the flower remedies will be suitable for you – whatever your mood.*

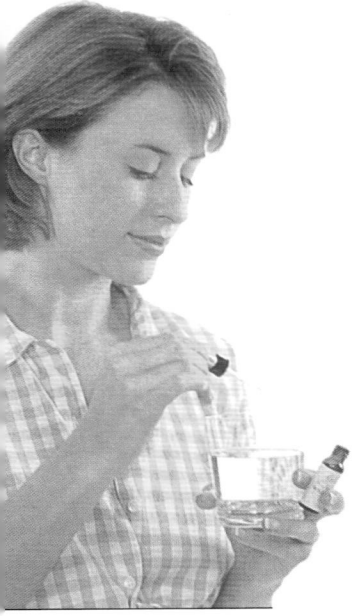

BACH REMEDIES FOR STRESS

Impatiens if you're energetic but tense.
Cherry plum if you're on the verge of a breakdown.
Clematis for absent-mindedness caused by withdrawal from the real world.
Rock rose for frozen terror and a sense of helplessness.
Star of Bethlehem for the after-effects of shock.
Agrimony for mental torment behind a brave face.
Aspen for fears of unknown origin.
Elm if overwhelmed by responsibility.
Gorse for despair.
Red chestnut when you're over-concerned for others.
Sweet chestnut for extreme mental anguish.
White chestnut for obsessive worrying.
Wild rose for apathy.

Spas & Beauty Therapy

Soothe Stresses Away In Luxury

Nothing is more soothing than being pampered. If you automatically think 'I can't do that – it costs too much', are you really broke? Or don't you feel right about 'wasting' money on pleasure for yourself? An occasional treat may not break the budget. Why not phone a few local places and find out?

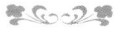

For some of us it's a hairdo – a gentle head massage and a flattering cut can do as much good as a holiday. And if your hairdresser makes you feel guilty about your split ends, go to someone else next time. Remember you're paying!

Others take refuge in beauty salons, which offer a wider range of comforts such as massage, pedicures, facials and body wraps. Again, it's the mixture of relaxation and beautifying which has such beneficial effects.

Some women don't like hands-on therapies, especially if they've had babies clambering over them all day. For them, a health club is the place. Don't bother with the sunbeds, they can damage your skin – head straight for the warmth and water.

Saunas put out an intense dry heat which some people love. But don't despair if it just brings your skin up in hot blotches – steam rooms are back in

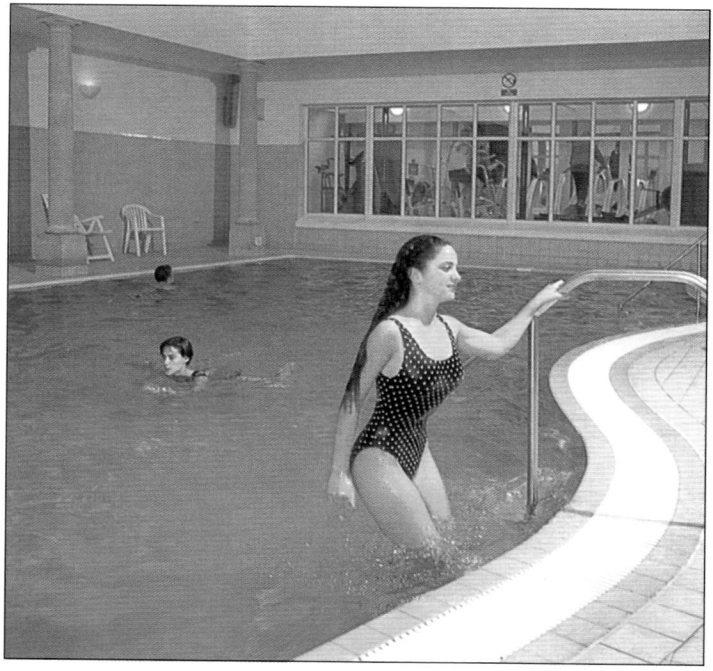

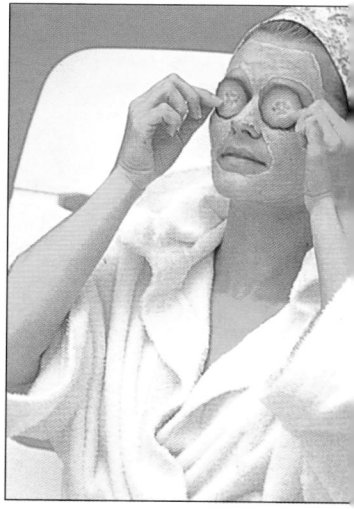

△ *Beauty treatments can be a real pick-me-up, making you look and feel great.*

◁ *A swim followed by a luxurious soak in the Jacuzzi is wonderfully relaxing.*

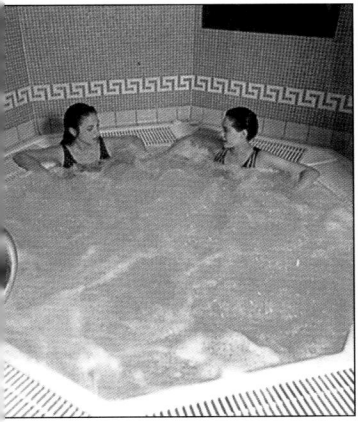

△ *Health clubs offer a variety of facilities for relaxation, including a Jacuzzi, steam room, sauna, as well as massage, reflexology, aromatherapy and beauty therapies.*

FLOAT TANK

You take a shower, then climb into a bathtub with a lid, or a tiny room like a flooded sauna, and shut yourself in. It's pitch dark and silent.

◆ You lie on water so salty that you float. Both water and air are at body temperature, so you can't feel anything. With nothing to stimulate your senses you may hallucinate.

And people do this willingly?

◆ Actually, it's astonishingly relaxing. You can turn the light on or scramble out whenever you like.

◆ Not everyone takes to it, but even claustrophobics find themselves letting go of the light cord and drifting peacefully in their own world.

◆ You may find beautiful or disturbing images well up from your unconscious. You may feel a deep sense of peace and oneness with the world. You may just get bored.

◆ Some centres play relaxing music and you can also bring a meditation or self-hypnosis tape – this is one place where you won't be distracted.

fashion now, hiding everyone in clouds of soft vapour. Then shower the sweat off and jump into the swimming pool or Jacuzzi. If you do all this after an aerobics class or game of tennis, of course, you'll have the added glow of virtue.

Are you going to a health resort? Congratulations! Shop around for one that meets your needs – some are real old-style fat farms, specialising in quick, short-term weight loss through hunger. Others are geared up for activity, and may help you start a fitness regime that's tailored to your needs.

If relaxation is your main aim, head for somewhere with treatments and facilities you would like to try, preferably in peaceful country surroundings. You could also contact health centres and retreats advertised in New Age magazines, which offer alternative therapies like crystal healing too.

▷ *Treat yourself to a beauty make-over, a hairdo or a facial – it will do wonders for your confidence.*

◆ If you're pregnant or suffer ill-health, especially a heart or skin condition, please check with your doctor before trying health club treatments. Don't use the float tank if you have mental health problems.

Bath Delights

Floating In Your Own World

Water is our element, just as much as air. It makes up 70 per cent of our bodies, and of the planet. Our long-ago ancestors evolved in warm seas, as we did in the waters of the womb. No wonder, that for most of us, sinking into a warm bath is the most relaxing moment of our day.

If you live alone, put the answering machine on or unplug the telephone. Otherwise, find a convenient time and let everyone know that you are not to be interrupted for, say, half an hour. If you have the place to yourself during the day, why not indulge in a luxurious afternoon soak? Treat yourself to some big, thick, fluffy towels and a bathrobe to snuggle into.

Then settle in for the most peaceful experience you could have. Make sure the room is warm, light some candles and turn off the overhead light. Put on a cassette of sea sounds or atmospheric relaxation music. For fragrance, use a scented candle or some aromatherapy oil in a burner.

Now's the time to cleanse your skin, smooth on some moisturizer or a facepack if you like and check the body lotion is at hand for when you step out. Add your

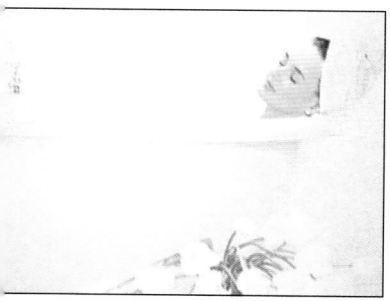

△ *Make sure you will not be disturbed and float off in your own private world.*

▷ *Listen to the sounds of summer in the garden – or play a tape to create the scene.*

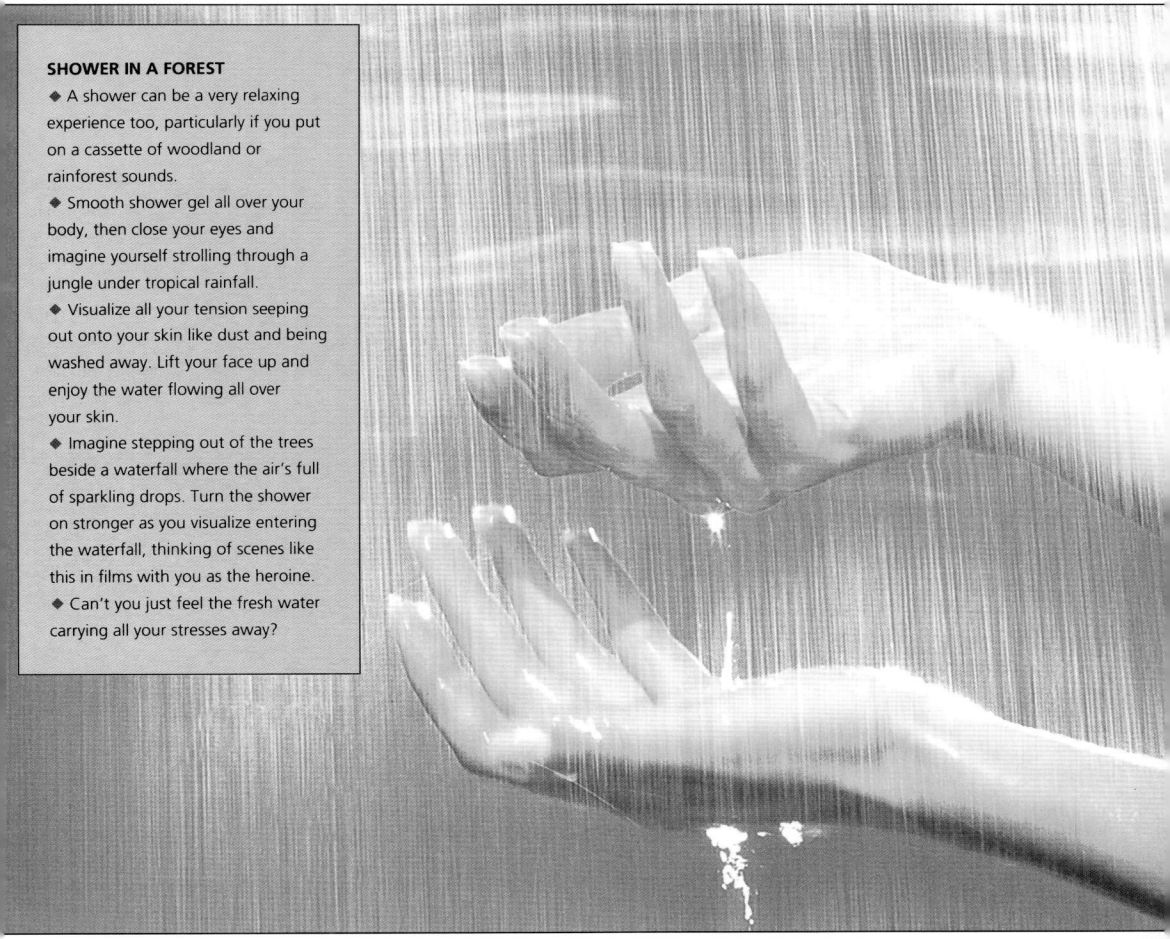

SHOWER IN A FOREST

◆ A shower can be a very relaxing experience too, particularly if you put on a cassette of woodland or rainforest sounds.

◆ Smooth shower gel all over your body, then close your eyes and imagine yourself strolling through a jungle under tropical rainfall.

◆ Visualize all your tension seeping out onto your skin like dust and being washed away. Lift your face up and enjoy the water flowing all over your skin.

◆ Imagine stepping out of the trees beside a waterfall where the air's full of sparkling drops. Turn the shower on stronger as you visualize entering the waterfall, thinking of scenes like this in films with you as the heroine.

◆ Can't you just feel the fresh water carrying all your stresses away?

favourite indulgences – foam bath under a running tap, essential oil just as you get in, a splash of your favourite cologne or a herbal treat you've made yourself. Then slip into the water and relax. This is a lovely time to do a foot-to-head relaxation or some affirmations.

Body heat

Water is said to have the most relaxing effects at body temperature – try it and see. If you don't have a thermometer, aim for a temperature at which you can't really tell if your hand's in the water or not when you test it. It may at first seem unpleasantly tepid, but persevere for at least 10 minutes, topping up with hot water to keep the temperature constant.

Otherwise, enjoy your bath warm rather than steaming. It's healthier, kinder to the skin, and more relaxing – very hot water has an exhausting effect.

◆ If you don't have a separate loo (with washbasin), it's worth putting that on your list of priorities next time you move house. As well as easing rush-hour pressure on the busiest room, it means no one has to use the bathroom while you're relaxing in it.

◆ Keep the cassette player a safe distance from any water.

Planning a Relaxation Day

A day at a health spa is something to save up for or put on your birthday wish-list. But with a bit of planning, a group of friends can organize their own relaxation day at little or no cost, using techniques from this book. With prerecorded tapes, you can even do it by yourself – or invite your best friend.

One person needs to be responsible for organizing, but she can still take part in most sections, using tapes where possible. (A psychological tip – people are much less likely to interrupt a tape.) Take the first few minutes of each section to make sure everyone knows what to do, and keep an eye on beginners in case they need help. At the end of the longer sessions, leave five minutes for people to stretch their legs and chat.

Everything should be at a comfortable level for newcomers to relaxation – remind them not to feel stressed if there's anything they can't manage. Oh, and make sure everyone has some idea about the methods you use, so no one fears meditation or yoga is the first step towards a satanic orgy!

If you're asking people to bring lunch to share, sort out who's bringing what so you don't end up with too many packs of identical cheese sandwiches or cakes. Aim for light, healthy food with plenty of fruit and salad, and provide a selection of herbal teas.

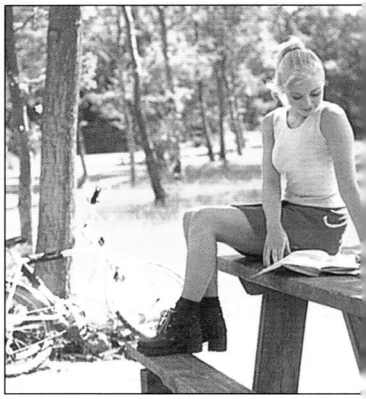

△ *Add your own ideas and favourite techniques for a tailor-made schedule.*

Use local resources if possible, do you know any trained people – a masseuse, reflexologist, yoga or t'ai chi teacher, for example – who'll give an hour of their time in return for lunch and taking part in the rest of the day? A local homeopath, herbalist or other alternative practitioner may also be willing to give a talk and demonstration.

If anyone suffers a health condition, especially epilepsy, high blood pressure or mental health problems, get them to check with their doctor that it's all right to join in.

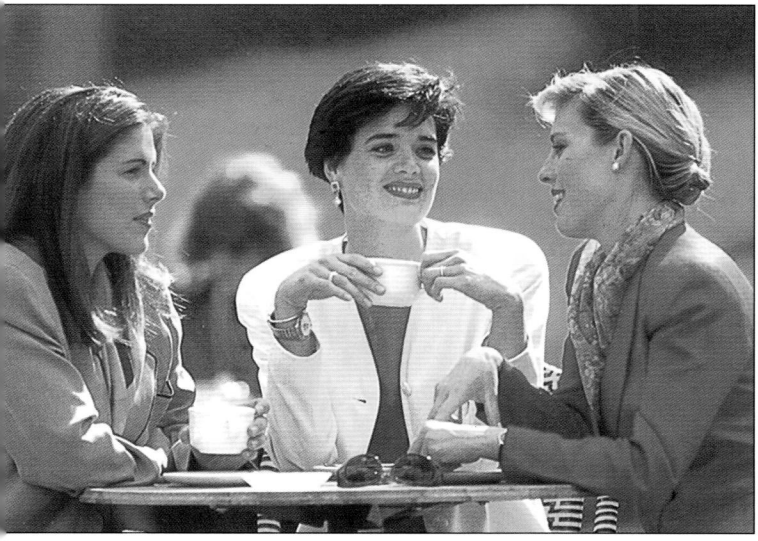

◁ *Why not invite your friends to a relaxation day? Perhaps they will share in the organizing and help to make tapes or volunteer their massage or yoga skills.*

WHAT YOU'LL NEED

- A quiet, empty room, big enough for everyone to lie on the floor. It's best with no one else in the house, so people won't feel inhibited or worry about what the kids are up to. Allow time to move furniture if necessary.
- A table or tray, access to hot water and a selection of herbal teas. Do include some decaffeinated coffee and ordinary tea though, for those who'd miss them too much to relax.
- Cushions, and straight-backed chairs for anyone who can't sit on the floor.
- A cassette recorder with peaceful background tapes such as New Age music or the sounds of the sea or woodland, plus dance music and Middle Eastern music for belly dancing.
- Notes or this book as back-up.

Optional:

- Oil if you're doing any massage.
- A tape to sing with.
- Candles and matches.
- Relaxing oils, a burner and spare nightlight candles.
- Pre-recorded cassettes for foot-to-head relaxation and meditation. If you do these 'live', write yourself a script in advance.
- Some spare blankets.
- A timer.

ASK PEOPLE TO BRING

- Lunch.
- Rainwear if the weather looks unreliable and some time is to be spent out of doors.
- A blanket to cover them while they're lying down.

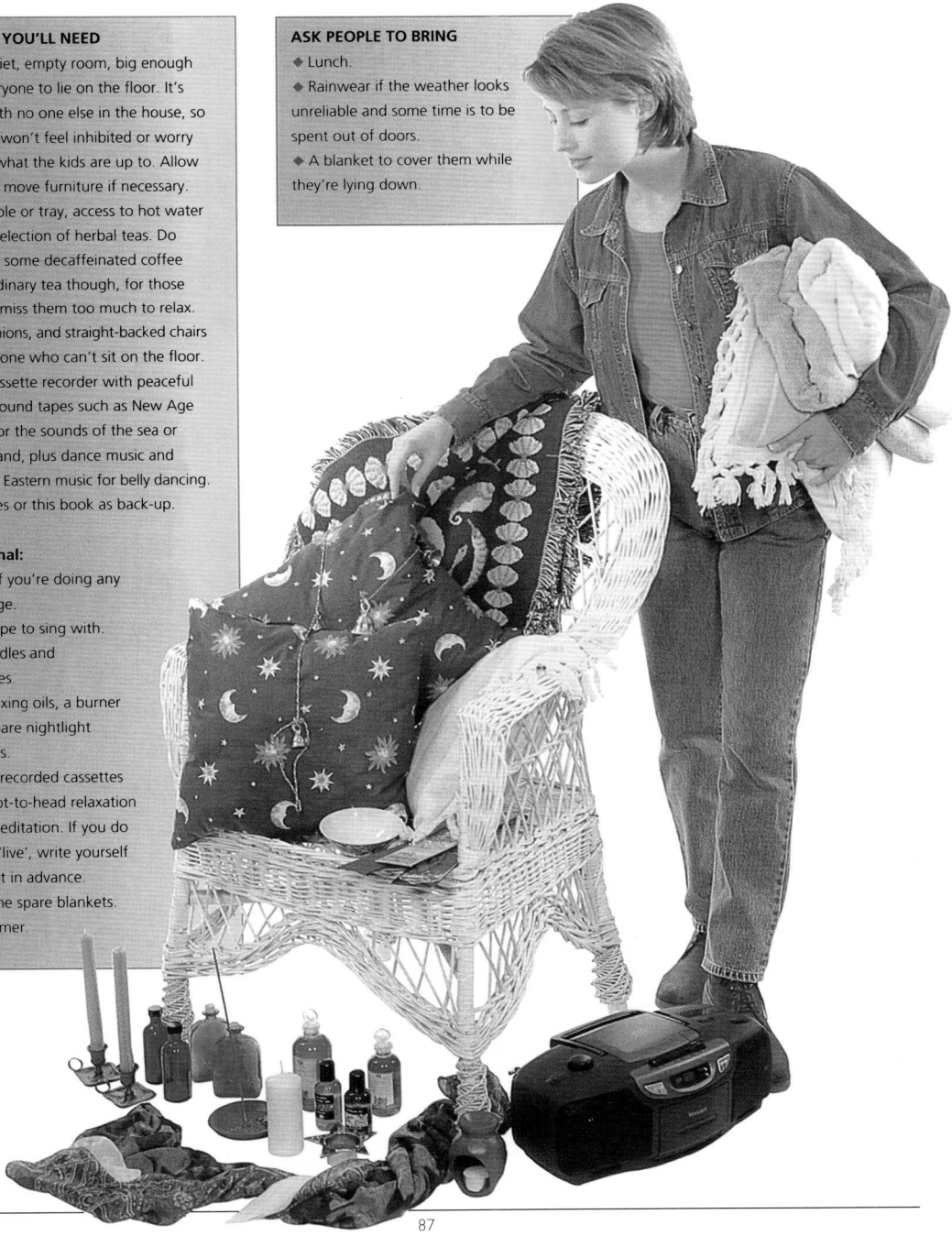

On The Day

For best results, organize a schedule for your relaxation day in advance and try to stick to it come what may. The timetable here, fitting round school hours, is just an example – you may want to work one out with the people who are going to take part.

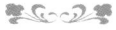

Are your friends sedentary workers who need more movement? Or exhausted young mothers who'd seize any chance of lying down? Would they like fewer, longer sessions, or a 10–5 day? Aim for variety without too many changes of pace, and remember not to schedule anything physically taxing straight after eating.

The important thing is not to let time dribble away in 'What shall we do next? ...'

Relaxation morning or evening

For a three-hour break, use the all-day timetable but leave out the period 12 – 2.39. In other words – focusing, breathing, meditation, stretch, belly dance and foot-to-head relaxation. If people are tired, replace the belly dance with voice therapy, moving meditation and yoga.

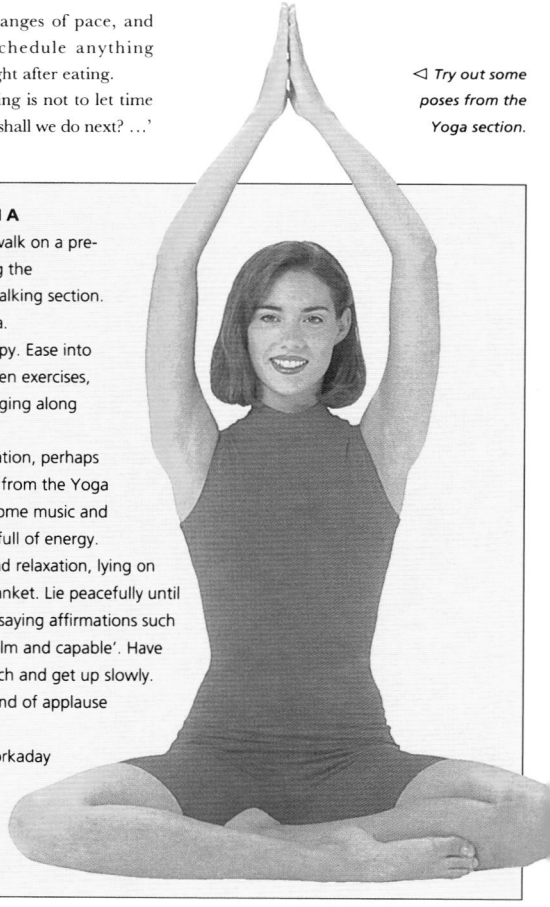

◁ Try out some poses from the Yoga section.

TIMETABLE – MORNING

9.30am Time for a cup of herbal tea while everyone arrives.

9.40am Focusing. Sit quietly in a circle for five minutes and get in the mood for the day. Then do some head and neck relaxers from page 30.

Move gently into:

9.50am Breathing exercises, ending with blue colour breathing.

And on to:

10am Seated meditation. Reassure newcomers that it doesn't matter if they don't feel they're meditating properly – just sitting peacefully is useful too.

10.30am Stretch session. Remind everyone to take it gently and never to do jerky movements.

11am Belly dancing – a change of pace with swirly Middle Eastern music – and probably lots of laughter! Wind down with a few minutes of Infinity meditation.

12 noon Lunch.

AFTERNOON PLAN A

12.30pm Go for a walk on a pre-planned route, using the techniques in the Walking section.

1.15pm Back for tea.

1.30pm Voice therapy. Ease into it with humming, then exercises, then chanting or singing along with a tape.

2pm Moving meditation, perhaps finishing with poses from the Yoga section. Or put on some music and dance if everyone's full of energy.

2.40pm Foot-to-head relaxation, lying on the floor under a blanket. Lie peacefully until 2.55, then finish by saying affirmations such as 'I am peaceful, calm and capable'. Have a long leisurely stretch and get up slowly.

2.59pm A huge round of applause for the organizer!

3pm Back to the workaday world, ready for anything.

Or, see afternoon plan B

AFTERNOON PLAN B – rain stops play

12.30pm Voice therapy.

1pm Massage. Pair people off to take turns massaging each other's neck and shoulders. If they'd like to try foot massage, demonstrate some simple kneading, squeezing and toe-pulling movements – a foot massage is so relaxing you don't need any brilliant techniques. Just remind everyone to avoid broken skin and to press hard enough not to tickle.

1.45pm Tea break.

2pm Continue as in Plan A.

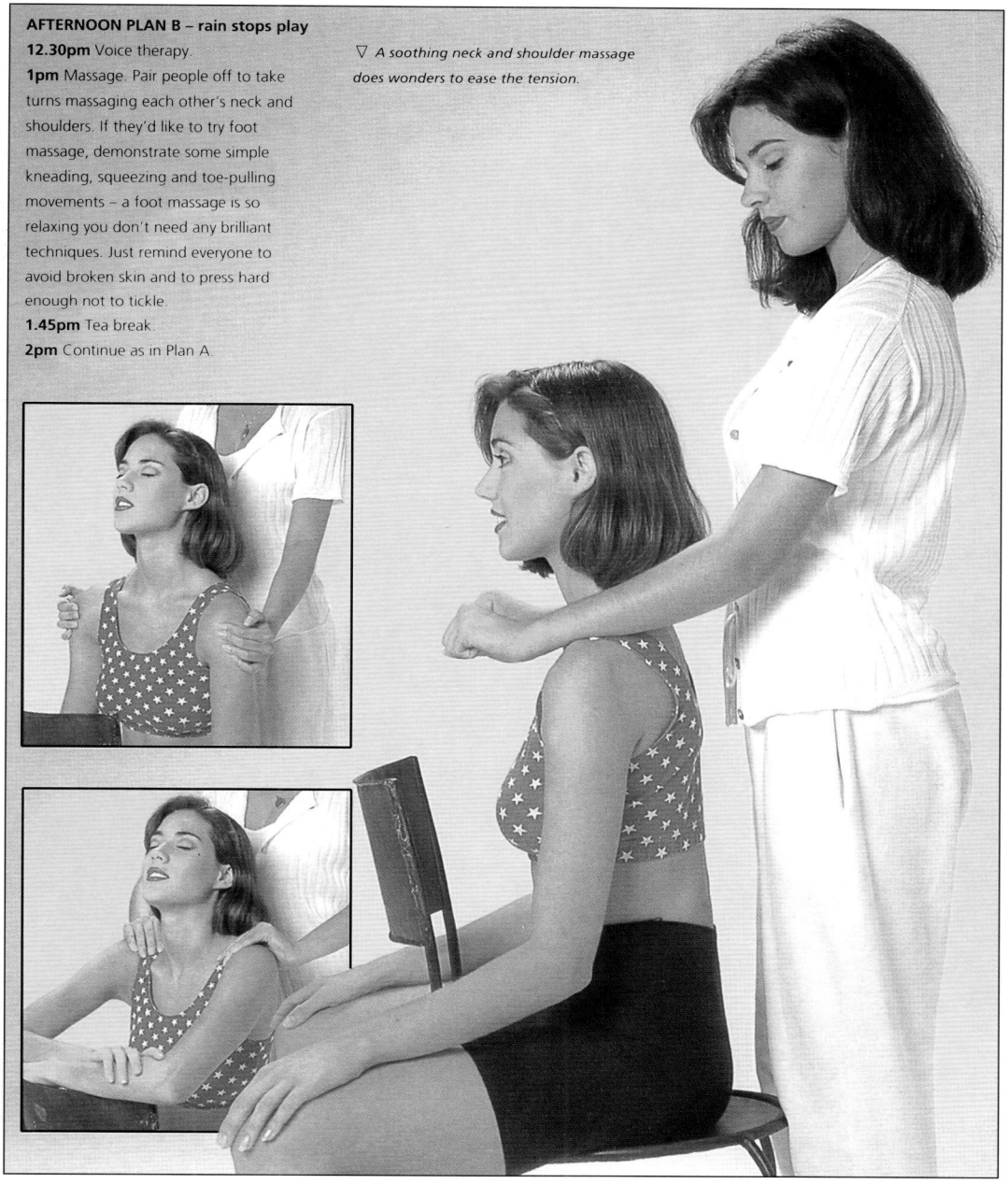

▽ *A soothing neck and shoulder massage does wonders to ease the tension.*

The Most Important Thing

All the techniques in this book are effective ways of reducing stress and increasing the ability to relax. It's a question of trying out some that appeal and finding which ones suit you. You'll probably end up with a repertoire of options for different situations.

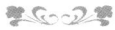

Don't forget the most important way of relieving stress – enjoying life. When you're overworked or weighed down with responsibilities, having fun slips a long way down the priority list. That's when you start grabbing at indulgences that don't even really give pleasure – stuffing food down, smoking without really noticing you're doing it, impulse-buying.

Instead, stop and think what you'd really enjoy doing. It doesn't have to be something you think is useful or a formal relaxation method.

If you're so out of the habit you can't think what you'd like, sit down quietly and wait for some options to float into your mind. A cafe meal with your best friend while the kids are at school? Swimming? Reading a novel in the park? Taking a bus to somewhere you've never been before? Going to bed? Taking a singing class? Then imagine yourself actually doing each of these things and spend a while noting how it feels.

Keep with it till you come up with something you can feel yourself enjoying. Then do it!

◆ Play games. Playing with children is one of the best ways to relax because you can do things their way – run, yell, laugh, fall down and roll on the grass. There's no better way of working off steam. No children around? Play with your partner or a friend. All you need is a football and someone to kick it around with.

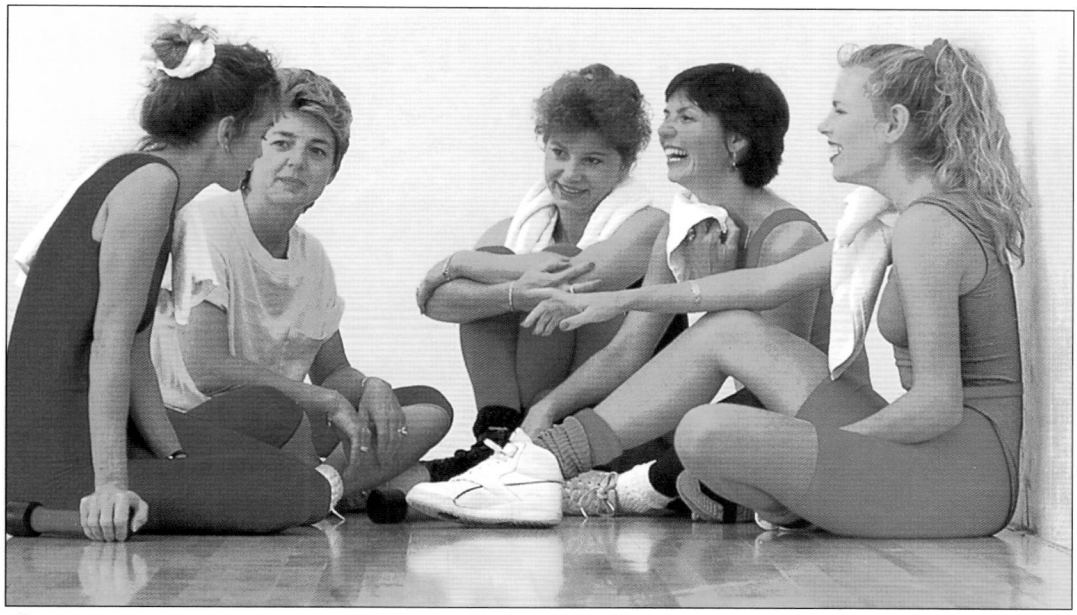

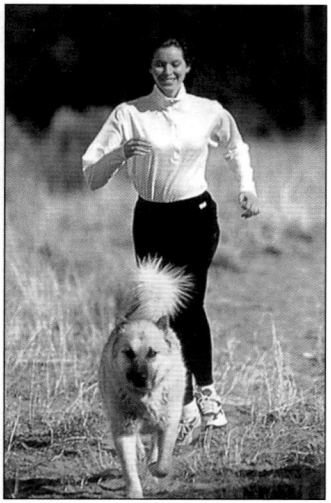

△ *Take a dog for a walk – or a run!*

◁ *Nothing is more fun than play.*

◆ Make a regular date with friends and take it in turns to organize something cheap and easy for fun.

◆ Take short breaks, like a weekend away or a day in the country. Longer holidays can sometimes be more stressful than relaxing, because of the organization and travelling involved – and because people feel under pressure to enjoy themselves.

◆ Spend time with your friends, but have things to do when you get some time to yourself to relax.

◆ Do something you don't usually do:

◆ Go to the ballet or theatre (tickets are often cheaper early in the week and at matinees).

◆ Fly a kite or borrow a pair of skates.

◆ Take someone's dog for a run.

◆ Get your friends together and go to a comedy club.

◆ Go bird-watching.

◆ Get your partner to join you on a long country walk ending in the pub.

△ *Going with friends helps you stay motivated and you can relax together afterwards.*

Bringing back the balance

If you're rushed and disorganized, the slowing relaxation techniques will help you make space in your life. Meditation and breathing exercises, in their various forms, are ideal.

If you tend to be very controlled, or get depressed and brood about problems, try some of the livelier techniques such as belly dancing or aerobics. Tune your radio to a pop station and do the wildest dance you've ever seen. Sing at the top of your voice (all right, start off quietly and work up). Run on the spot for a minute, then turn the movement into a silly dance.

Shopping to Relax

You don't need any equipment at all to relax. But if you feel like treating yourself or starting a birthday list, the items on these pages were created to aid relaxation.

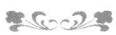

Health food shops are a good place to start – they stock books, essential oils and all kinds of relaxation aids as well as food. With more people taking an interest in alternative healing, pharmacies too may sell homeopathic medicines, flower remedies and essential oils. Department stores have many of the electrical items. And health and beauty shops stock all kinds of massage-related goods.

To burn oil you can buy candle-fuelled pottery burners from craft stalls and health food shops, or larger electric versions from department stores. Another handy little electric gadget is a negative ionizer, which many people find refreshes the air.

To help with massage, there's a vast range of sophisticated electric devices that knead your muscles tirelessly. Nowadays there's so much choice – vibrating hairbrushes, cushions, chairs, beds, you name it – that it's worth trying out different models. At the simple end of the scale are small, low-cost wooden rollers that do a similar job with muscle power.

Even if you don't suffer from back ache, specialist back-care shops and catalogues have a lot of comfortable furniture and other items – apart from aiding relaxation now, they could prevent back problems starting. Chinese and novelty shops may stock pairs of metal balls with tiny bells inside, to roll in one hand with tranquillizing effects. Wind chimes and indoor fountains can create a peaceful ambience too.

Feet get such a bad deal in everyday life that they come in for a lot of special treatment in the relaxation world. Look out for massage sandals, spiky rollers, vibrating electric pads, miniature whirlpools and all kinds of potions to rub into them. No more than they deserve.

But the kindest thing you can do for your feet, or your back, is to sink into a Banana Chair. This extraordinary-looking device is one of the most comfortable pieces of furniture ever made – you simply lie in it with your feet up, perfectly supported, then put on some peaceful music and drift away.

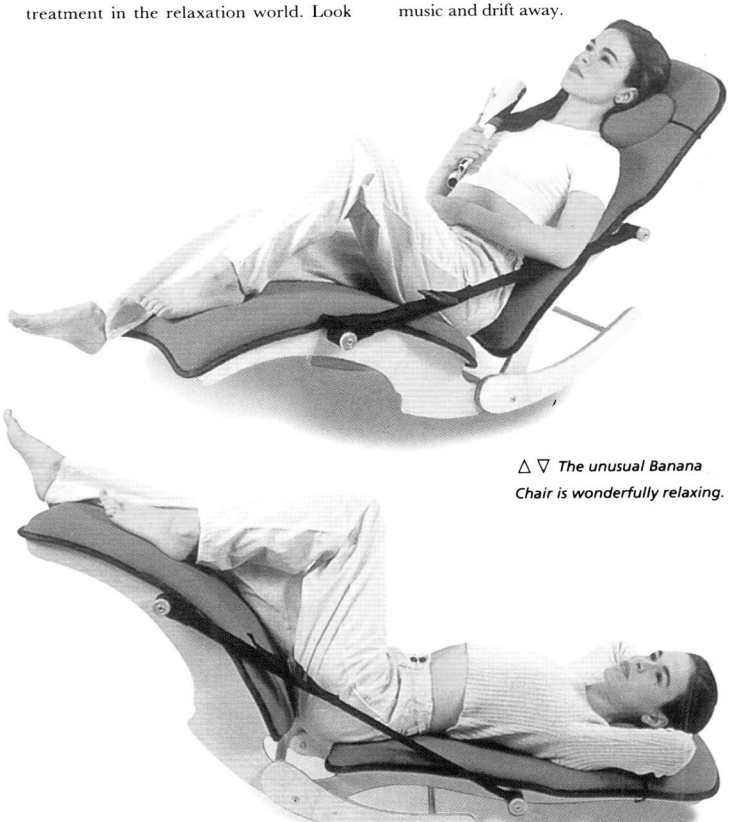

△ ▽ *The unusual Banana Chair is wonderfully relaxing.*

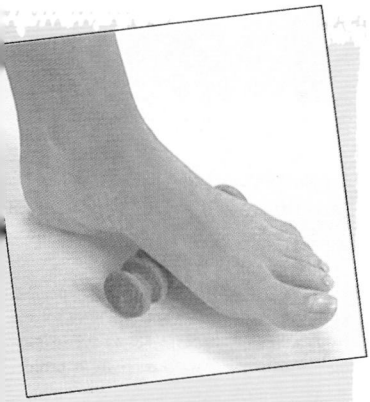

△ *Look out for treats for your feet.*

Relaxation tapes are now so widely available that you can take your pick of styles, accents, with or without music, from a variety of shops or by mail order. There are all kinds of variations on the muscle-relaxation theme, with accompanying visualizations.

The same is true for hypnotherapy tapes, covering stress-relief as well as giving up smoking, gaining confidence and just about anything else you could want to do. One popular series is by British hypnotherapist Jean Credland, whose reassuring, down-to-earth voice makes the whole process feel wonderfully natural. Her *Rainbow Meditation* tape uses colour imagery, as does American Nancy Hopps's *Relaxation/Affirmation Techniques*.

The same shops and catalogues tend to sell relaxing music tapes and CDs, including ambient, ethnic and sounds from nature. Lose yourself in some tribal drumming for moving meditation, or join in with chanting Tibetan monks.

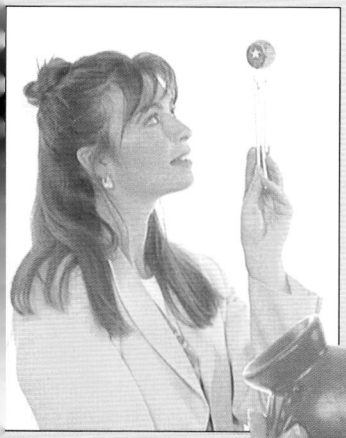

△ *Wind chimes can create a peaceful ambience.*

> *Check out health shops, craft shops, pharmacies and department stores to discover a wide variety of different products to help you unwind.*

Where Do I Go From Here?

The safest way to find a local practitioner is through personal recommendation or by sending an SAE to a reputable organization, including those mentioned on these pages.

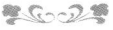

It is especially important to take care with hypnotherapy or hands-on treatments, which could be harmful if done incorrectly. Ask the practitioner in advance about costs and what the treatment involves.

Unlike doctors or nurses, alternative practitioners don't legally have to know anything about their subject. Anyone can set up a training school or award meaningless qualifications, so letters after people's names may not always be a sign of expertise.

People often visit alternative practitioners when they're going through a bad patch. In situations like that it's easy for an unscrupulous person to take advantage, or convince people they should do whatever the 'expert' says. It's rare, but it has happened, so if you feel uncomfortable just leave.

For more information about various therapies, send a stamped, self-addressed envelope to:

◆ **The Institute for Complementary Medicine**, PO Box 194, London SE16 1QZ, UK, tel 0171-237 5165 (SAE and two loose stamps). Practitioners of various alternative therapies can take an ICM exam, marked by independent assessors. If successful, they can join the British Register of Complementary Practitioners and put the letters BRCP after their name in addition to their existing qualification.

◆ **The British Complementary Medicine Association**, 39 Prestbury Road, Pittville, Cheltenham, Glos GL52 2PT, UK tel: 01242 226770.

◆ **The Australian Traditional Medicine Society**, PO Box 422, Ryde, New South Wales 2112, Australia, tel: 02 809 6800.

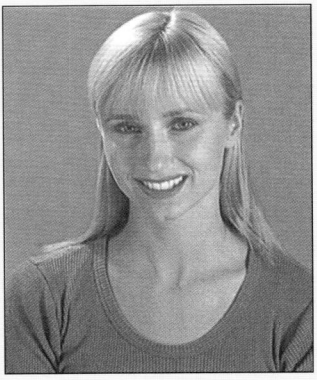

◆ **American Holistic Medical Association**, 4101 Lake Boone Trail, Ste 201, Raleigh NC 27607, tel: (919) 787 5181.

◆ *Holistic Health Directory,* published by New Age Journal (address right) lists US practitioners state by state.

STANDING UP TO STRESS
Smokers' Quitline, tel 0171-487 3000.
The Council for Involuntary Tranquillizer Addiction, Cavendish House, Brighton Road, Waterloo, Liverpool 22 5NG, UK, tel 0151-949 0102. An international service offering advice and information.
The National Council for Voluntary Organisations, Regents Wharf, 8 All Saints Street, London N1 9AL.
The Health Address Book, from **The Patients' Association**, 18 Victoria Park Square, London E2 9PF, tel 0181-981 5676. Lists every UK self-help group you could think of.

PMS
Women's Nutritional Advisory Service, PO Box 268, Lewes, East Sussex BN7 2QN, UK, tel 01273 487366.
Beat PMS Through Diet by Maryon Stewart (Vermilion).

PEACEFUL PREGNANCY
Healthy Parents, Healthy Baby by Maryon Stewart (Headline).

RELAX? WITH KIDS LIKE MINE?
Hyperactive Children's Support Group, 71 Whyke Lane, Chichester, West Sussex PO19 2LD, UK, tel 01903 725182.
Mothers and Others for a Livable Planet, 40 W 20th Street, New York NY 10011, tel (212) 242 0010.

MOVING WITH THE CHANGE
Breezing through the Change by Ellen Brown and Lynne Walker (Frog Ltd).
The Pause by Lonnie Barbach (Bantam).

COPING WITH PAIN
Pain Wise UK, 33 Kingsdown Park, Tankerton, Kent CT5 2DT, UK, tel 01227 277886.
Pain Relief Foundation, Rice Lane, Walton, Liverpool L9 1AE, UK, tel 0151-523 1486. Information including mail order relaxation and pain-relief audio tapes. Send large SAE.

ORGANIZE TO AVOID STRESS
How to Make Life Easy for Yourself by Denise Katz (Angus and Robertson).
LETSLINK UK, Liz Shepherd, c/o 61 Woodstock Road, Warminster, Wiltshire BA12 9DH, UK. Information about alternative currencies; organized schemes to barter goods and services.

TAKING IT FROM THE TOP
Eva Fraser's Facial Workout (Penguin).

MASSAGE
The Book of Massage by Lucinda Lidell (Ebury).
The Massage Manual by Fiona Harrold (Headline).
American Massage Therapy Association, 820 Davis Street, Suite 100, Evanston, IL 60201, US, tel (708) 864 0123.
Associated Bodywork and Massage Professionals, 28677 Buffalo Park Road, Evergreen CO 80439-7347, tel (303) 674-8478.

SELF-MASSAGE
Self-Massage by Monika Struna and Connie Church (Vermilion).
Self-Massage by Jacqueline Young (Thorsons).

SHIATSU

The Art of Shiatsu by Oliver Cowmeadow (Element).
Do-It-Yourself Shiatsu by Wataru Ohashi (Unwin).

AROMATHERAPY

International Federation of Aromatherapists, Stamford House, 2–4 Chiswick High Road, London W4 1TH, UK. Send £2 and A5 SAE.
International Federation of Aromatherapists, 25 Singleton Road, North Baldwyn, Victoria 3104, Australia.
National Association for Holistic Aromatherapy, PO Box 17622, Boulder, Colorado 80308-6799, US.
The Aromatherapy Organisations Council, 3 Latymer Close, Braybrooke, Market Harborough, Leics LE16 8LN, UK, tel 01858 434242.
Aromatherapy: an A–Z by Patricia Davis (CW Daniel UK).
Aromatherapy by Julie Sadler (Ward Lock).
Aromatherapy and the Mind by Julia Lawless (Thorsons).

REFLEXOLOGY

Association of Reflexologists, 27 Old Gloucester Street, London WC1, UK, tel 0181-451 2218.
International Institute of Reflexology, PO Box 12642, St Petersburg, FL 33733, tel (813) 343 4811.
Reflexology: Foot Massage for Total Health by Inge Dougans with Suzanne Ellis (Element).
Step by Step Reflexology by Renee Tanner (Douglas Barry Publications 21 Laud Street, Croydon, Surrey CR0 1SU, UK).

ALEXANDER TECHNIQUE

North American Society of Teachers of the Alexander Technique, PO Box517, Urbana IL 61801, tel (800) 473 0620.
Alexander Technique by Chris Stevens (Optima).
Body Know-How by Jonathan Drake (Thorsons).

YOGA

The Yoga Biomedical Trust, UK, tel 01223 67301.
Yoga Therapy by Stella Weller (Thorsons).
Yoga for Common Ailments by Drs R Nagarathna, HR Nagendra and Robin Monro (Gaia).

T'AI CHI

Tai Chi by Danny Connor (Stanley Paul).
Infinite Tai Chi video by Jason Chan from Talking Pictures, PO Box 77, Cirencester, Glos GL7 5YN, UK.

EXERCISE

Exercise Association, Unit 4 Angel Gate, City Road, London EC1V 2PT, UK, tel 0171-278 0811. Qualified instructors.
Sports Council, 16 Upper Woburn Place, London WC1H 0QP, UK, tel 0171-388 1277.
American Council on Exercise, 5820 Oberlin Drive, Suite 102, San Diego, California 92121-3787, US, tel 619 535 8227.
Fitness Industry Association, PO Box 60, Arncliffe, New South Wales 2205, Australia, tel 02 264 9699.
Keep Moving! It's Aerobic Dance by Esther Kan and Minda Goodman Kraines (Mayfield).
Health & Fitness magazine, Nexus House, Azalea Avenue, Swanley, Kent BR8 8HY, UK, tel 01322 660070.

STRETCH

The Complete Book of Stretching by Tony Lycholat (Crowood UK).

BELLY DANCE

Belly Dancing for Health and Relaxation by Tina Hobin (Duckworth UK).
Sorra Enterprises, The White Cottage, High Street, Harwell Village, Oxon OX11 0EX, UK, tel 01235 834073. Music tapes, costumes, books and information on classes.

AUTOGENIC TRAINING

The British Association for Autogenic Training and Therapy, 18 Holtsmere Close, Watford, Herts WD2 6NG, UK.
Autogenic Training by Dr Kai Kermani (Thorsons).

MEDITATION

Meditation for Everybody by Louis Proto (Penguin).
Meditation, a Treasury of Technique by Pam and Gordon Smith (CW Daniel).
The Everyday Meditator by Osho (Boxtree).

MINDFULNESS

Ad Brugman, The Orchard, Lower Maescoed, Hereford HR2 0HP, UK, tel 01873 860207. Runs mindfulness courses.
The Experience of Insight by Joseph Goldstein (Unity Press).
The Miracle of Mindfulness by Thich Nhat Hanh (Beacon).

MOVING MEDITATION

The Everyday Meditator by Osho (Boxtree).
The Serpent and the Wave by Jalaja Bonheim (Celestial Arts).
Raven Recordings, 744 Broad Street, Room 1815, Newark, New Jersey 07102, US, tel (201) 642 7942 and Raven Recordings, Staccato, Bridam, Kents Road, Wellswood, Torquay TQ1 2NN, UK, tel 01803 295442. Music tapes and videos by Gabrielle Roth, guru of modern meditation.
Susannah and Ya'Acov, Darling Khan, 01803 762255. Five to Midnight, Nappers Crossing, Staverton, South Devon TQ9 6PD, UK. Moving meditation.

SELF-HYPNOSIS

Self-Hynosis by Valerie Austin (Thorsons).

COLOUR THERAPY

The Book of Colour Healing by Theo Gimbel (Gaia Books).
Susan Farrar, The Iris Centre, 10 Princes Road, London SW14 8PE, UK, tel 0181-876 2548.

VOICE THERAPY

Susan Lever, 2 Woodlea, Coulby Newham, Middlesbrough TS8 0TX, UK, tel 01642 590562. Workshops, sound healing and voice therapy tapes.
Frankie Armstrong, 45 Cecil Street, Cardiff CF2 1NW, UK, tel 01222 480429. Singing and voice workshops.
Mim Beim, Sydney, Australia, tel (02) 211 3811. Naturopathy and voice work.
Voice Movement Therapy Association, PO Box 4218, London SE22 0JE, UK.
The Book of Sound Therapy by Olivea Dewhurst-Maddock (Gaia).

HERBALISM

The National Institute of Medical Herbalists, 56 Longbrook Street, Exeter, Devon EX4 6AH, UK.
The General Council and Register of Consultant Herbalists, Marlborough House, Swanpool, Falmouth, Cornwall TR11 4HW, UK.
Baldwin & Co, 171 Walworth Road, London SE17 1RW, UK. Herbal supplier.
The Herb Society's Home Herbal by Penelope Ody (Dorling Kindersley).
Herbal Healing for Women by Rosemary Gladstar (Bantam).
The Herbal for Mother and Child by Anne McIntyre (Element).

HOMEOPATHY

The British Homeopathic Association, 27a Devonshire Street, London W1N 1RJ, UK, tel 0171-935 2163. (Medically qualified homeopaths.)
The Society of Homeopaths, 2 Artizan Road, Northamptom NN1 4HU, UK, tel 01604 21400. (Lay homeopaths.)
The Complete Guide to Homeopathy by Dr Andrew Lockie and Dr Nicola Geddes (Dorling Kindersley).
Homoeopathy: Heart and Soul by Dr Keith Souter (CW Daniel).
Homoeopathic First Aid by Dr Anne Clover (Thorsons).

FLOWER REMEDIES

International Federation for Vibrational Medicine, Middle Piccadilly Natural Healing Centre, Holwell, nr Sherborne, Dorset DT9 5LW, UK, tel 01963 23468.
The Dr E Bach Centre, Mount Vernon, Sotwell, Wallingford, Oxon OX10 0PZ, UK, tel 01491 834678.
International Flower Essence Repertoire, The Working Tree, Milland, Liphook, Hants, GU30 7JS, UK, tel 01428 741672. Remedies by mail order.
Nelson Bach USA, Dept NJ95, 1007 West Upsal Street, Philadelphia PA 19119, US, tel 1-800-314 BACH.
The Australian Flower Remedy Society, PO Box 531, Spit Junction, New South Wales 2088, Australia.
The Encyclopaedia of Flower Remedies by Clare G Harvey and Amanda Cochrane (Thorsons).

SPA AND BEAUTY THERAPY

Healthy Venues, UK, tel 01203 690300. Bookings for many health resorts, including treatments.
Spa Finders, US, tel (212) 924 7240. Bookings for health resorts.

SHOPPING

Banana Chair Company, Unit 10, Langley Park, North Street, Langley Mill, Notts NG16 4BS, UK, tel 01733 533626.
Jean Credland, Rainbows, 7 Baile Hill Terrace, York YO1 1HF, tel 01904 629024.
Nancy Hopps, Synergistic Systems, PO Box 5224, Eugene, OR 97405, US, tel (503) 683 9088.
Deep Wave Music, The Womad Shop, 3 George Centre, Crewkerne, Somerset TA18 7JW, tel 01460 77444. Mail order.
New World Cassettes, Paradise Farm, Westhall, Halesworth, Suffolk IP19 8RH, UK. Mail order.
New World Productions, PO Box 244 WBO, Red Hill, Queensland 4059, Australia, tel (07) 367 0788. Mail order music.
Alternative View, The Old Auction Mart, Station Approach, Godalming, Surrey GU7 1EW, UK, tel 01483 415225. Mail order videos.
Mysteries, 9 Monmouth Street, London WC2H 9DA, UK, tel 0171-240 3688. Shop and mail order, many relaxation items.
Educating Hands Bookstore, 261 SW 8th Street, Miami, Florida 33130, US, tel (305) 285 0651. Shop and mail order books, tapes, videos and more.
Quintessential Oils, 847 35th Street, Richmond CA94805, US. Massage and herbal products.

AND MORE...

All kinds of treatments, goods, holidays, workshops and mail order catalogues are advertised in magazines such as:
Kindred Spirit, Foxhole, Dartington, Totnes, Devon TQ9 6EB, tel 01803 866686.
New Age Journal, 42 Pleasant Street, Watertown MA 02172, US, tel (617) 926 0200.
Australian WellBeing, Freepost 3, PO Box 249, Mosman, NSW, Australia 2088, tel (02) 969 7122.

Index

affirmations *20, 56, 84, 88.*
alcohol *8, 16, 80.*
back 12, *18, 28, 30, 32, 34, 36, 38, 44, 46, 48, 54, 58, 92.*
breathing *8, 9, 18, 20, 28, 48, 54, 56, 62, 66, 72, 74, 90.*
children *6, 7, 8, 10, 12, 14, 16, 24, 42, 46, 56, 72, 74, 90.*
coffee *8, 16, 22, 76, 78, 86.*
confidence *20, 72, 74, 92.*
dancing *10, 52, 58, 66, 74, 90.*
depression *10, 12, 16, 52, 72, 76, 90.*
driving *6, 56, 64, 74.*
energy (strength and vitality) *6, 7, 9, 10, 16, 22, 24, 58, 60, 68, 80.*
enjoyment *7, 16, 24, 52, 64.*
exhaustion *7, 10, 14, 40, 78, 84.*
face *7, 14, 20, 30, 32, 38, 84.*
fear *12, 16, 18, 78, 80, 86.*
feet *18, 20, 26, 32, 34, 38, 40, 44, 46, 48, 50, 54, 56.*
food *6, 8, 10, 14, 16, 22, 24, 64, 78, 80, 86, 88, 90.*
fun *16, 20, 58, 72, 90.*
hands *28, 30, 34, 36, 38, 40, 44, 46, 50, 64, 66, 70, 78, 92.*
happiness *56, 70, 72, 90.*
headaches *10, 20, 38, 40, 42, 44, 74, 76, 78.*
herbs *8, 14, 20, 40, 76, 84, 86.*
hormones *6, 10, 12, 16, 22, 28, 48, 52.*
life force, *see Energy*
muscles *7, 8, 18, 20, 30, 32, 34, 36, 38, 44, 46, 54, 58, 60, 68, 72, 74, 92.*
oils *10, 12, 14, 22, 26, 36, 42, 44, 72, 84, 86, 92.*
slimming diets *22.*
smoking *12, 14, 64, 68, 90, 92.*
tea *8, 22, 86.*
tranquillizers *8, 76.*
visualization *18, 26, 70, 72, 84, 92.*
water *9, 14, 56, 64, 76, 82, 84, 86.*

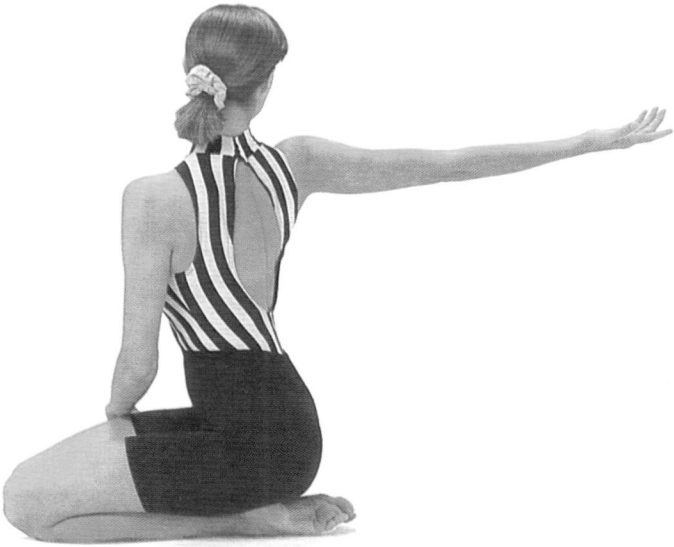